W9-BXV-983

The Washington Manual™ Allergy, Asthma, and Immunology Subspecialty Consult

The Washington Manual™ Allergy, Asthma, and Immunology Subspecialty Consult

Faculty Advisor
Daniel Hamilos, M.D.
Associate Professor of Medicine
Washington University School of Medicine
St. Louis, Missouri

The Washington Manual™ Allergy, Asthma, and Immunology Subspecialty Consult

Editors

Barbara Capes Jost, M.D.
Fellow, Division of Allergy and Immunology
Department of Medicine
Washington University School of Medicine
Barnes-Jewish Hospital
St. Louis Children's Hospital
St. Louis, Missouri

Khaled M. Abdel-Hamid, M.D., Ph.D.
Allergist, private practice
St. Louis, Missouri

Elizabeth C. Friedman, M.D.
Genessee Health Service, Allergy,
Rheumatology, and Immunology
Rochester, New York

Alpa L. Jani, M.D.
Fellow, Division of Allergy and Immunology
Department of Medicine
Washington University School of Medicine
Barnes-Jewish Hospital
St. Louis, Missouri

Series Editor

Tammy L. Lin, M.D.
Adjunct Assistant Professor of Medicine
Washington University School of Medicine
St. Louis, Missouri

Series Advisor

Daniel M. Goodenberger, M.D.
Professor of Medicine
Washington University School of Medicine
Chief, Division of Medical Education
Director, Internal Medicine Residency Program
Barnes-Jewish Hospital
St. Louis, Missouri

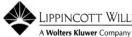

LIPPINCOTT WILLIAMS & WILKINS
A **Wolters Kluwer** Company
Philadelphia · Baltimore · New York · London
Buenos Aires · Hong Kong · Sydney · Tokyo

Acquisitions Editor: Danette Knopp
Developmental Editors: Scott Marinaro and Keith Donnellan
Supervising Editor: Allison Risko
Production Editor: Lucinda Ewing, Silverchair Science + Communications
Manufacturing Manager: Colin Warnock
Cover Designer: QT Design
Compositor: Silverchair Science + Communications
Printer: RR Donnelley

Library of Congress Cataloging-in-Publication Data

The Washington manual allergy, asthma, and immunology subspecialty consult / [edited by] Barbara Capes Jost ... [et al.].
    p. ; cm. -- (The Washington manual subspecialty consult series)
  Includes bibliographical references and index.
  ISBN 0-7817-4374-5
  1. Allergy--Handbooks, manuals, etc. 2. Asthma--Handbooks, manuals, etc. 3. Immunology--Handbooks, manuals, etc. I. Title: Allergy, asthma, and immunology subspecialty consult. II. Jost, Barbara Capes. III. Series.
  [DNLM: 1. Hypersensitivity--diagnosis--Outlines. 2. Hypersensitivity--therapy--Outlines. WD 300 W319 2003]
  RC585.W37 2003
  616.97--dc21

2003044667

The Washington Manual™ is an intent-to-use mark belonging to Washington University in St. Louis to which international legal protection applies. The mark is used in this publication under license from Washington University.

Care has been taken to confirm the accuracy of the information presented and to describe generally accepted practices. However, the authors, editors, and publisher are not responsible for errors or omissions or for any consequences from application of the information in this book and make no warranty, expressed or implied, with respect to the currency, completeness, or accuracy of the contents of the publication. Application of this information in a particular situation remains the professional responsibility of the practitioner.

The authors, editors, and publisher have exerted every effort to ensure that drug selection and dosage set forth in this text are in accordance with current recommendations and practice at the time of publication. However, in view of ongoing research, changes in government regulations, and the constant flow of information relating to drug therapy and drug reactions, the reader is urged to check the package insert for each drug for any change in indications and dosage and for added warnings and precautions. This is particularly important when the recommended agent is a new or infrequently employed drug.

Some drugs and medical devices presented in this publication have Food and Drug Administration (FDA) clearance for limited use in restricted research settings. It is the responsibility of health care providers to ascertain the FDA status of each drug or device planned for use in their clinical practice.

10 9 8 7 6 5 4 3 2 1

Contents

Contributing Authors

Khaled M. Abdel-Hamid, M.D., Ph.D.

Allergist, private practice
St. Louis, Missouri

Gregg J. Berdy, M.D., F.A.C.S.

Instructor in Clinical Ophthalmology
and Vision Science
Department of Ophthalmology
Instruction and Research
Washington University
School of Medicine
St. Louis, Missouri

Susan S. Berdy, M.D.

Assistant Professor of Clinical Medicine
Department of Medicine
Washington University
School of Medicine
St. Louis, Missouri

Elizabeth C. Friedman, M.D.

Genessee Health Service, Allergy,
Rheumatology, and Immunology
Rochester, New York

Anne C. Graff

Barnes-Jewish Hospital
St. Louis, Missouri

Mitchell Grayson, M.D.

Instructor in Medicine
Washington University
School of Medicine
St. Louis, Missouri

Alpa L. Jani, M.D.

Fellow, Division of Allergy and
Immunology
Department of Medicine
Washington University
School of Medicine
Barnes-Jewish Hospital
St. Louis, Missouri

Shirley S. Joo, M.D.

Chief Resident
Clinical Instructor
Washington University
School of Medicine
Barnes-Jewish Hospital
St. Louis, Missouri

Barbara Capes Jost, M.D.

Fellow, Division of Allergy and
Immunology
Department of Medicine
Washington University
School of Medicine
Barnes-Jewish Hospital
St. Louis Children's Hospital
St. Louis, Missouri

Diane R. Klueppel

Barnes-Jewish Hospital
St. Louis, Missouri

Robin G. Lorenz, M.D., Ph.D.

Associate Professor
Department of Pathology
University of Alabama at Birmingham
Birmingham, Alabama

Jennifer McKay

Barnes-Jewish Hospital
St. Louis, Missouri

Jill A. Poole, M.D.

Fellow-in-Training, Department of
Allergy, Asthma, and Immunology
National Jewish Medical and
Research Center
Denver, Colorado

Chairman's Note

Medical knowledge is increasing at an exponential rate, and physicians are being bombarded with new facts at a pace that many find overwhelming. The Washington Manual™ Subspecialty Consult Series was developed in this context for interns, residents, medical students, and other practitioners in need of readily accessible practical clinical information. The series therefore meets an important need in an era of information overload.

I would like to acknowledge the authors who have contributed to these books. In particular, Tammy L. Lin, M.D., Series Editor, provided energetic and inspired leadership, and Daniel M. Goodenberger, M.D., Series Advisor, Chief of the Division of Medical Education in the Department of Medicine at Washington University, is a continual source of sage advice. The efforts and outstanding skill of the lead authors are evident in the quality of the final product. I am confident that this series will meet its desired goal of providing practical knowledge that can be directly applied to improving patient care.

Kenneth S. Polonsky, M.D.
Adolphus Busch Professor
Chairman, Department of Medicine
Washington University
School of Medicine

Series Preface

The Washington Manual™ Subspecialty Consult Series is designed to provide quick access to the essential information needed to evaluate a patient on a subspecialty consult service. Each manual includes the most updated and useful information on commonly encountered symptoms or diseases and highlights the practical information you need to gather before formulating a plan. Special efforts have been made to organize the information so that these guides will be valuable and trusted companions for medical students, residents, and fellows. They cover everything from questions to ask during the initial consult to issues in subsequent management.

One of the strengths of this series is that it is written by residents and fellows who know how busy a consult service can be, who know what information will be most helpful, and who can detail a practical approach to patient care. Each volume is written to provide enough information for you to evaluate a patient until more in-depth reading can be done on a particular topic. Throughout the series, key references are noted, difficult management situations are addressed, and appropriate practice guidelines are included. Another strength of this series is that it was written in concert. All of the guides were designed to work together.

The most important strength of this series is the collection of authors, faculty advisors, and especially head authors assembled to write this series. In addition, we received incredible commitment and support from our chairman, Kenneth S. Polonsky, M.D. As a result, the extraordinary depth of talent and genuine interest in teaching others at Washington University is showcased in this series. Although there has always been house staff involvement in editing The Washington Manual™ series, it came to our attention that many of them also wanted to be involved in writing and making decisions about what to convey to fellow colleagues. Remarkably, many of the head authors became junior subspecialty fellows while writing their guides. Their desire to pass on what they were learning, while trying to balance multiple responsibilities, is a testament to their dedication and skills as clinicians, teachers, and leaders.

We hope this series fulfills the need for essential and practical knowledge for those learning the art of consultation in a particular subspecialty and for those just passing through it.

Tammy L. Lin, M.D., Series Editor
Daniel M. Goodenberger, M.D., Series Advisor

Preface

This is the first edition of The Washington Manual™ Subspecialty Consult Series, born out of a long tradition of excellence in the form of *The Washington Manual of Medical Therapeutics*, now in its 30th edition. The series, written by residents in the Department of Medicine and fellows in the subspecialties of the Department of Medicine, is primarily for use by interns, residents, medical students, and primary care practitioners. We think that it may also be a practical, concise tool for fellows-in-training and a sound reference tool for ancillary medical staff.

This manual of Allergy, Asthma, and Immunology is designed to be a timely resource outlining current concepts and practice guidelines in this rapidly evolving and exciting field.

We are grateful for the guidance and careful review of our manuscript by Dr. Daniel Hamilos, our faculty advisor. We would like to thank Dr. Mitchell Grayson for his thoughtful and timely comments on our manuscript. With gratitude, we acknowledge also Dr. Hamsa Subramanian, who provided excellent feedback during the early stages of our manuscript. In addition, we are proud to have had the editorial assistance of a fine group of faculty members and personal mentors: Dr. H. James Wedner, Dr. Phillip E. Korenblat, Dr. J. Allen Thiel, Dr. Rand Dankner, Dr. Talal Chatila, Dr. Peter Tuteur, Dr. John Wood, Dr. Helena Schotland, Dr. Mike Walter, and Dr. Robin Lorenz.

B.C.J.
K.M.A
E.C.F.
A.L.J.

Key to Abbreviations

ACE	angiotensin-converting enzyme
AIDS	acquired immunodeficiency syndrome
ANCA	antineutrophil cytoplasmic antibody
ASA	aspirin
BP	blood pressure
CBC	complete blood count
CHF	chronic heart failure
CNS	central nervous system
COPD	chronic obstructive pulmonary disease
CT	computed tomography
CVA	cardiovascular accident
DNA	deoxyribonucleic acid
ELISA	enzyme-linked immunosorbent assay
ER	emergency room
ESR	erythrocyte sedimentation rate
FDA	U.S. Food and Drug Administration
FEV_1	forced expiratory volume in 1 second
GI	gastrointestinal
HEENT	head, ears, eyes, nose, throat
HIV	human immunodeficiency virus
HLA	human leukocyte antigen
HTN	hypertension
ICU	intensive care unit
Ig	immunoglobulin
NSAID	nonsteroidal antiinflammatory drugs
OR	operating room
PEF	peak expiratory flow rate
RAST	radioallergosorbent assay test
RBC	red blood cell
WBC	white blood cell

1

Approach to the Allergic Patient

Mitchell Grayson

HISTORY

The single most important component in diagnosing allergic disorders is taking a full and complete history. Important elements:

- **Symptoms:** Fully explore the types of symptoms and when and how often they occur.
- **Exacerbating/alleviating factors:** What makes the patient's symptoms worse? What makes them better? Does exposure to pets, smoke, perfume, or a change in air temperature affect them? Are certain seasons better than others?
- **Environmental history:** Often overlooked, it may be critical in determining an occupational allergy exposure. Where does the patient work, live, and play? What exposures are present in each of these environments? Does the patient have a pet? Does the pet have access to the patient's bedroom?
- **Family history:** Allergic diseases have a strong hereditary link. Therefore, it is important to find out if there are other members of the family with allergic diseases. A child with one parent with allergic disorders has a 40% chance of having allergies (being atopic). Having two parents with allergic disorders increases the risk to 60–80%.
- **Psychosocial issues:** Often, a failed interaction with a patient results from unanticipated or identified psychosocial barriers. Be aware of these issues and understand the patient's goals for the clinic visit.

DIAGNOSTIC TESTS

Because of the risk of false-positives with all testing modalities, all positive results must be correlated with clinical sensitivity.

Skin Testing

The most rapid and specific methods to test for allergic sensitivity, these tests are based on mast cell degranulation due to the patient's skin's being exposed to specific allergens. Because the read-out of these tests depends on the release of histamine from mast cells, *antihistamines will block the effects of skin testing and must be discontinued before testing*. Two types of skin tests exist (see Chap. 8, *In Vivo* and *In Vitro* Diagnostic Tests for Allergy).

Epicutaneous Tests

- Most specific test available, but less sensitive than intradermal testing.
- Identifies most clinically significant allergens.
- Only method that should be used for food allergens.

Intradermal Tests

- More sensitive than epicutaneous, but less specific (therefore, many more false-positives).
- Increased risk of a systemic reaction.

In Vitro Tests (RAST Testing)

In vitro tests are designed to screen for the presence of allergen-specific IgE in the patient's serum by using immobilized allergen on a solid phase. Because these tests rely on IgE in the blood, and not mast cell degranulation, they may give positive results for allergens to which patients are not being exposed and from which they are not having symptoms. In general, the sensitivity and specificity of *in vitro* tests are similar to those of intradermal tests (see Chap. 8, *In Vivo* and *In Vitro* Diagnostic Tests for Allergy).

KEY COMPONENTS OF THE PHYSICAL EXAM

Appearance

* Due to nasal congestion, the patient may be mouth breathing.
* The patient may have allergic shiners, dark regions under the eyes due to nasal tissue edema, which compresses the draining veins under the eyes.
* Infraorbital folds or Dennie's lines may be present.
* A transverse line across the lower portion of the nose or nasal crease may be present. It is caused by the "allergic salute" patients give when they rub upward across their nose with the palm of the hand.

Skin Exam

* **Urticaria**, or hives, is a maculopapular erythematous eruption in the cutaneous tissues and is often quite pruritic.
* Edema of the subcutaneous tissues, or angioedema, is often painful but not pruritic.
* The tendency to form wheal and flare responses (urticate) to firm pressure applied to the skin is known as **dermographism**. Patients with dermographism may have physical urticarias causing their recurrent skin rashes.
* Check for dry, scaly patches on the extensor surfaces of the limbs. This is often **atopic dermatitis** and is associated with allergic diseases.

HEENT

Evaluate nasal anatomy. It is critical to look in the nares for swollen and edematous turbinates, polyps (whitish to clear sacs often hanging from the underside of the turbinates), and any septal deviation, ulceration, or perforation that may alter airflow.

Pulmonary

A thorough lung exam is required, including auscultation of the lung fields to listen for any evidence of wheezing or an increased expiratory phase. In some patients, when wheezing cannot be heard at rest, the use of a forced expiratory maneuver may be helpful.

KEY POINTS

* A well-organized and thorough history is critical in diagnosing allergic diseases.
* Diagnostic evaluation with skin testing or RAST testing to determine allergic sensitivities must be correlated with clinical symptoms.
* The physical exam should be directed toward the major target organs of allergic disease; in particular, the skin, HEENT, and pulmonary exams are most important.

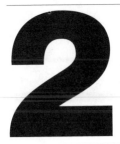

Basic Immunology Underlying Allergic Reactions and Allergic Inflammation

Jennifer McKay

INTRODUCTION

Immediate hypersensitivity is the hallmark of allergic disease and encompasses disorders such as asthma, anaphylaxis, and allergic rhinitis. Central to this process are mast cells and IgE. This chapter provides a brief overview of the immunology underlying allergic reactions and allergic inflammation.

MAST CELLS

Mast cells are metachromatic effector cells found near portals of entry, including lung and skin, that are critical for both innate and acquired defense mechanisms. They associate with blood vessels and nerves as well as inflammatory and malignant foci and are most notable for their abundant cytoplasmic granules and mediators that are released by immune and nonimmune stimuli. They are stimulated through the surface high-affinity receptor for IgE, termed *FcεRI*. Antigen binding and cross-linking of cell surface–bound IgE result in mast cell degranulation and activation. This interaction is what drives hypersensitivity and atopic reactions.

Developing Mast Cells

Developing mast cells arise from $CD34^+$ bone marrow progenitors. Maturation and granule acquisition occur in the periphery near blood vessels.

Mast Cell Granules

Mast cell granules contain several **preformed mediators**, enzymes, and cytokines, including histamine, chymase, heparin, tryptase, and tumor necrosis factor alpha (TNF-alpha), that are released within minutes of cross-linking of surface-bound IgE. **Newly formed mediators**, including lipid mediators, made through the lipoxygenase pathway (Table 2-1) are synthesized *de novo* at the time of mast cell activation. They have various effects, including vasodilation, increasing vascular permeability, and potentiating smooth muscle spasm.

Histamine
Histamine increases vascular permeability and causes smooth muscle contraction and vasodilation. Clinically, histamine mediates pruritus, increases airway secretions, and causes the cutaneous wheal and flare reaction.

Tryptase
Tryptase is a neutral protease and major granule component that has several forms:

- The constitutively secreted alpha isoform. Blood levels of alpha-tryptase are indicative of overall mast cell numbers and are markedly increased in patients with mastocytosis.
- The beta isoform. Blood levels of beta tryptase are normally quite low. It is released primarily during mast cell degranulation and therefore is a marker of a recent mast cell

TABLE 2-1.   NEWLY FORMED MEDIATORS OF THE ALLERGIC RESPONSE

IL-4, IL-13	Promote IgE isotype switching
	IL-13 promotes bronchial hyperresponsiveness
TNF-alpha	Promotes leukocyte recruitment into sites of allergic inflammation by inducing expression of cellular adhesion molecules on vascular endothelium
IL-5	Stimulates eosinophilopoiesis
IL-6	Stimulates B-cell differentiation
LTC_4, LTD_4	Potent bronchoconstrictors
	Increase vascular permeability
	Promote mucus hypersecretion and mucosal edema
TxA_2, PGD_2	Vasoconstrictor and bronchoconstrictor
PAF	Platelet aggregation, neutrophil and eosinophil chemotaxis, bronchoconstriction, peripheral vasodilation

degranulation event. Blood levels typically peak within 30–120 mins after an anaphylactic reaction but may persist above baseline levels for 6–12 hrs after the inciting event.

Newly Formed Mediators

Newly formed mediators, such as leukotrienes (LTC_4, LTD_4, LTE_4), prostaglandin D_2 (PGD_2), platelet activating factor (PAF), and cytokines, such as TNF-alpha, are synthesized *de novo* after mast cell degranulation.

- Their effects are seen in both the early and late phases of allergic reactions.
- Cytokines contribute primarily to late-phase allergic reactions (see Table 2-1). Cytokine-dependent mechanisms are thought to be a bridge between mast cell activation by IgE and subsequent late-phase reactions that result in inflammatory cell recruitment. This leads to ongoing inflammation followed by tissue damage and other changes found in chronic allergic disorders.

Stimuli for Mast Cell Degranulation

Stimuli for mast cell degranulation include

- Allergens, via cross-linking of surface IgE molecules.
- Antibodies that bind IgE or the FcεRI receptor and result in cross-linking.
- Various histamine-releasing factors, including certain members of the chemokine family, such as MIP-1α and neuropeptides, including substance P.
- Other secretagogues, including complement components (anaphylatoxins), drugs (morphine, codeine), and IV contrast dye.
- Physical stimuli, including pressure, heat, cold, and sunlight.

Clinical Effects

Clinical effects produced by mast cell mediators include urticaria, angioedema, eczema, rhinitis, conjunctivitis, asthma, laryngeal edema, and anaphylaxis (see Chap. 13, Anaphylaxis).

Anaphylaxis

- **Immediate allergic response:** The reaction begins when IgE already bound to mast cells via its high-affinity receptor (FcεRI) is cross-linked by an antigen. This stimulates the immediate release of mast cell granules containing preformed mediators such as tryptase, chymase, and histamine. These early-phase mediators cause local and systemic reactions within minutes of mast cell degranulation and last for up to an hour.

- **Late-phase allergic response**: The late-phase response (LPR) is mediated in part by newly formed lipid mediators (including PGD_2, PAF, and leukotrienes $LTC_4/D_4/E_4$) produced by mast cells and basophils. Inflammatory cells and cytokines (see Table 2-1) also mediate the LPR. Inflammation, the hallmark of the late-phase reaction, begins hours after the initial stimulus and may last for days. Cytokines released by mast cells during the immediate allergic response, such as IL-4 and TNF-alpha, stimulate expression of adhesion molecules on endothelial cells. Adhesion molecule expression plus elaboration of other chemokines allow for transendothelial migration of inflammatory cells into sites of allergic inflammation. Key infiltrating inflammatory cells include CD4 T lymphocytes, basophils, and eosinophils.
- Immediate and late-phase allergic responses have been described in several organs, including the lungs, nasal mucosa, conjunctiva, and skin. The mechanisms underlying these responses are similar in each organ.

IgE

IgE is a 190-kd immunoglobulin that exists in minute concentrations in the serum. It does not activate the complement pathway, nor is it involved in opsonization and neutralization of antigens. Mechanistically, its activity occurs through its interaction with IgE receptors located on mast and other cells of the immune system. More specifically, IgE's interaction via high-affinity (FcεRI) receptors on mast cells begins a cascade of events collectively described as *type I hypersensitivity*.

Serum IgE

Serum IgE is often found in higher concentrations in allergic individuals, but measurement of serum IgE has very limited clinical value.

Biological Activity

Biological activity of IgE occurs by interacting with receptors found on mast cells, basophils, and, to a lesser extent, Langerhans' cells, dendritic cells, and monocytes.

High-Affinity Receptor

The high-affinity receptor (FcεRI) has three subunits. The alpha subunit binds the ligand. The beta and gamma subunits are required for signal amplification and transduction, respectively.

- The FcεRI on monocytes and dendritic and Langerhans' cells does not have the beta subunit–amplification component.
- Mast cell degranulation occurs when a threshold level of antigens binds and cross-links surface-bound IgE molecules.
- IgE binding causes the FcεRI to be up-regulated, making it require smaller numbers of antigens for mast cell activation. Therefore, individuals with higher concentrations of IgE will likely require a smaller stimulus for mast cell activity to occur.

Low-Affinity Receptor (FcεRII)

The low-affinity receptor (FcεRII) is a single-chain transmembrane protein with two isoforms.

- The **A isoform** is found on B cells, and the **B isoform** is found on B cells, T cells, monocytes, and eosinophils.
- **FcεRII** mediates cytotoxic responses by monocytes, macrophages, platelets, and eosinophils and is able to down-regulate its own expression.

TABLE 2-2. HYPERSENSITIVITY REACTIONS

Type	Mechanism	Examples
I	IgE-mediated mast cell degranulation and activation	Allergic rhinitis, anaphylaxis, acute urticaria, atopic dermatitis, food allergy, insect sting allergy, allergic asthma
II	IgG or IgM binds antigen on cell surface, causing phagocytosis or complement-mediated cellular destruction	Autoimmune or drug-induced hemolytic anemia, Rh incompatibility, Goodpasture's disease
III	Immune complex–mediated disease	Serum sickness, hypersensitivity pneumonitis, SLE, vasculitis
IV	Delayed-type hypersensitivity (T-cell mediated)	Tuberculin reaction, allograft rejection, graft-vs-host disease, contact dermatitis

IgE Synthesis

IgE synthesis is regulated by a complex pathway that causes B cells to differentiate into IgE-producing cells. B cells require IL-4 to undergo isotype switch to produce IgE. The IL-4 is a "helper signal" derived from $CD4^+$ Th2 helper T lymphocytes.

- Antigen presentation to T cells usually results in a low-grade inflammatory process whereby IgG is produced by B cells. This is accomplished when the T-cell activation response to an antigen involves the secretion of gamma-interferon (gamma-IFN) and IL-2. This T-cell activation/differentiation pathway is called the **Th1 pathway**.
- When a macrophage engulfs an antigen by phagocytosis or pinocytosis, it begins to secrete IL-12. This promotes the differentiation of activated T lymphocytes toward the Th1 phenotype, resulting in the production of gamma-IFN.
- In the atopic individual, antigen presentation to T cells results in the production of cytokines such as IL-4, IL-5, and IL-13 that promote the production of IgE. This is called the **Th2 pathway**.
- During development, immunologic priming occurs via the placenta. Once a baby is born, its response to antigens is predominately of the Th2 pathway. In the nonatopic individual, the immunologic response normally shifts toward primarily the Th1 phenotype. Genetics and the environment both determine which pathway will dominate.

HYPERSENSITIVITY REACTIONS

Hypersensitivity reactions are well described in the medical literature and are an essential part of basic pathology. They are mechanisms by which the immune system causes injury to tissues. Normally, an antigen encountered by various cells of the immune system stimulates an inflammatory response that protects the body from the environment. Inflammation, therefore, is both protective and damaging. Hypersensitivity reactions describe the many ways that tissue damage can occur. Table 2-2 describes these reactions according to the classification by Gell and Coombs.

KEY POINTS

- Cross-linking of IgE molecules anchored on mast cells by antigen **triggers mast cell degranulation, mediator release, and *de novo* synthesis** of lipid-derived mediators.
- The **immediate allergic response** is mediated by mast cells, whereas the **late-phase allergic response** is mediated by other inflammatory cells, including CD4 T lymphocytes, basophils, and eosinophils.

- The **Th1 pathway** is characterized by the production of IL-12 and gamma-IFN. The **Th2 pathway** results in the production of IL-4, IL-5, and IL-13 and production of IgE.

SUGGESTED READING

Costa JJ, Weller PF, Galli SJ. The cells of the allergic response. *JAMA* 1997;278(22):1815–1822.

Kay AB. Allergy and allergic diseases—first of two parts. *N Engl J Med* 2001;344(1):30–37.

Middleton CE, Reed EF, Ellis NF, et al., eds. *Allergy: principles and practice*, 5th ed. St. Louis: Mosby, 1998.

Allergic Rhinitis and Sinusitis

Jennifer McKay

ALLERGIC RHINITIS

Introduction

Allergic rhinitis is a common condition characterized by rhinorrhea, nasal congestion, postnasal drainage, nasopharyngeal itching, and sneezing. It is the clinical manifestation of tissue changes in the upper airway in response to IgE-specific interactions leading to mast cell degranulation. Its hallmark is the temporal relationship between onset of symptoms and exposure to antigens, such as dust mites or pollens. This history is often difficult to obtain because of the many other conditions that can mimic allergic rhinitis. Allergic rhinitis is thought to affect 10–20% of the population. Most people with allergic rhinitis develop the disease before age 20 and have a family history of allergic disease.

Causes

Mechanism
When an inhaled allergen comes in contact with allergen-specific IgE-sensitized basophils and mast cells located superficially in the mucosa of the respiratory tract, the mast cells degranulate. This causes release of preformed mediators and, later, newly synthesized mediators, which are responsible for the early and late phases of an allergic reaction (see Chap. 1, Approach to the Allergic Patient).

Differential Diagnosis
The differential diagnosis is lengthy but can be divided into two categories: allergic and nonallergic.

ALLERGIC RHINITIS

Definition. *Allergic rhinitis* is defined as allergen-driven mucosal inflammation. More specifically, it is the clinical manifestation of IgE-specific interactions with mast cells. It can be seasonal, perennial, or occupational. The key to diagnosis is that symptoms occur in a temporal relationship with allergen exposure.

Symptoms. Symptoms of watery rhinorrhea, itching, and sneezing during times when pollen counts are high, as in the spring or fall, are consistent with allergic rhinitis. Waxing and waning of symptoms with the seasons are typical of this condition; however, because of late-phase effects, symptoms can persist beyond the pollen seasons. Patients may have associated symptoms of allergic conjunctivitis (itchy, watery eyes), and pruritus of the palate or ear canals. Occasionally, patients complain of reduced sense of smell (hyposmia or anosmia), but the presence of this symptom should alert the clinician to the possible presence of chronic sinusitis or nasal polyposis, or both.

Perennial allergic rhinitis is defined as symptoms for >2 hrs/day for >9 mos of the year. This condition results from chronic exposure to molds, pet danders, or dust mites. Perennial allergic rhinitis is often associated with seasonal exacerbations.

NONALLERGIC RHINITIS. *Nonallergic rhinitis* is defined as inflammation of nasal mucosa that is not mediated by IgE. Many conditions are associated with this finding:

- **Infectious rhinitis** is acute or chronic, and its etiologies include bacteria, fungi, and viruses. Viruses are the most common cause. History should suggest a recent upper respiratory infection. Symptoms include fever, facial pain or pressure, purulent discharge, decreased sense of smell, and cough. The most common bacterial causes are *Streptococcus pneumoniae*, group A beta-hemolytic *Streptococcus*, and *Haemophilus influenzae*. If the patient is severely immunocompromised, one should consider opportunistic fungal infections.
- **Vasomotor rhinitis** is chronic nasal congestion secondary to excessive vasomotor activity. The cause is unknown, but nonimmune stimuli may play a role in mast cell degranulation. Odors, alcohol, spicy foods, emotions, temperature change, and bright light are known triggers of this problem.
- **Drugs** are frequently incriminated in causing rhinitis, and the most common offenders are antihypertensives, including ACE inhibitors and beta-blockers, as well as aspirin, NSAIDs, oral contraceptives, and cocaine. **Samter's triad** is the occurrence of aspirin sensitivity, nasal polyps, and asthma.
- **Nonallergic rhinitis with eosinophilia syndrome (NARES)** is very similar to allergic rhinitis, but skin tests to specific allergens are negative.
- **Nasal polyps** are pale, smooth, round, gelatinous-appearing outgrowths from the nasal passages usually beginning on the lateral nasal wall that are often confused with enlarged nasal turbinates. They contain eosinophils and immunoglobins with eosinophil-associated growth factors likely responsible for their growth. The presence of nasal polyps in children should alert one to the possibility of cystic fibrosis.
- **Hormonal rhinitis** is associated with nasal obstruction and hypersecretion in conjunction with hypothyroidism, pregnancy, or oral contraceptive use. In pregnancy, symptoms often develop in the second trimester and remit upon delivery.
- **Anatomic causes** include choanal atresia, adenoid hypertrophy, tumors, foreign bodies, and septal deviation.

Presentation

History and Physical Exam
A history of seasonal watery rhinorrhea, sneezing, itching, and nasal congestion is typical of allergic rhinitis. Given the long list of conditions that mimic it, a thorough history is important. One should note specific triggers; medication lists; environmental conditions, including whether pets or carpets are present in the home; and family history of atopy. Physical exam often reveals a transverse crease across the bridge of the nose secondary to persistent upward rubbing (the "allergic salute"), Dennie's lines (folds inferior to the lower lid), conjunctivitis, and allergic shiners (periorbital darkening). Careful evaluation of nasal passages is important for ruling out nasal polyps or anatomic abnormalities, such as septal deviation, tumors, and foreign bodies.

Management

Lab Analysis and Imaging
Skin testing is recommended to confirm the diagnosis of allergic rhinitis and to identify specific allergenic triggers. Skin testing also is used to guide treatment if immunotherapy is needed (see Treatment). Skin tests for aeroallergans are less expensive, more specific, and more clinically relevant than RAST (see Chap. 8, *In Vivo* and *In Vitro* Diagnostic Tests for Allergy) in allergic rhinitis. Serum IgE may be elevated in patients with allergic rhinitis but is frequently normal; therefore, it should not be used as a diagnostic aid. The presence of eosinophils in nasal cytology helps to differentiate between allergic and infectious rhinitis, but nasal cytology is not often done. When clinically appropriate, CT scanning should be used to rule out structural causes or associated sinusitis (see Sinusitis). Indications for CT are the presence of chronic sinusitis not responding to therapy, acute recurrent sinusitis, and persistent facial pain.

Treatment

Minimizing exposure to allergens by **environmental modification** is important for reducing symptoms. Patients should be instructed to close windows and doors during pollen season, use occlusive bedding for mattresses and pillows, avoid contact with pets, and wear a face mask when allergens cannot be avoided.

Intranasal steroids are effective at preventing the early and late phases of an allergic reaction and are the mainstay of therapy. For patients with known seasonal allergic rhinitis, the best results occur when intranasal steroids are begun 1 wk before pollen season's onset. There are numerous intranasal steroids on the market. Systemic side effects are minimal; however, patients should be instructed on their proper use to prevent nasal septum trauma. A meticulous examination of the nasal passages for evidence of septal ulceration and, rarely, perforation is important once nasal steroids have been prescribed, and they should be discontinued if epistaxis occurs repeatedly.

Antihistamines reduce symptoms of rhinorrhea, nasal pruritus, sneezing, ocular pruritus, and tearing and may reduce nasal congestion. Second-generation antihistamines come in nonsedating preparations. Avoid the use of sedating first-generation antihistamines in the treatment of allergic rhinitis.

Nasal decongestants, such as pseudoephedrine (Actifed, Allercon, Allerfrim, Allerfrin, Histafed) and phenylephrine (Despec-SF, Neo-Synephrine), decrease nasal congestion but should be used at the lowest effective dose. Side effects include insomnia, headache, palpitations, and tachycardia. Judicious use of intranasal decongestants is important, because rebound congestion occurs if used >5–7 days. During this time, tachyphylaxis and, later, nasal hypertrophy that appears clinically as beefy, red mucosa develop. This condition is known as **rhinitis medicamentosa**. Oral decongestants may be used chronically in selected patients. Side effects include insomnia, headache, palpitations, and tachycardia.

Oral steroids are rarely indicated in the treatment of allergic rhinitis because of systemic side effects.

Cromolyn sodium is a mast cell stabilizer that is somewhat effective in reducing sneezing, itching, and rhinorrhea.

Montelukast, a leukotrine-receptor antagonist, was recently approved for treatment of seasonal allergic rhinitis.

Immunotherapy is used to treat perennial and seasonal rhinitis when a specific allergen has been identified. Most often, immunotherapy is used when medical management and environmental controls have failed. Immunotherapy is successful approximately 80% of the time and should be considered unsuccessful if the patient has no relief from symptoms after 1 yr of maintenance therapy. One should also consider discontinuing immunotherapy after 3–5 yrs in patients who have responded well to the treatment. Immunotherapy is the only treatment modality that alters the natural history of the disease. Its sucess requires careful patient selection.

SINUSITIS

Introduction

Background

Sinusitis is closely associated with rhinosinusitis and often occurs secondary to local processes after viral infections. Most often, it is caused by infection. Clinical characteristics are facial pain and pressure, nasal congestion, purulent discharge, cough, postnasal drainage, headache, and pain in the upper teeth. Cough may be especially bothersome. It is a common chronic condition that has significant impact on health care. It constitutes up to 20% of office visits to allergists and accounts for many missed workdays. It is, however, a challenge for physicians to treat and often is referred on to surgeons when medical treatment has failed.

Definition

Sinusitis is inflammation of one or more of the paranasal sinuses and is classified as acute, chronic, and recurrent. Although there are no consensus standards defining chronic vs acute sinusitis, it is generally accepted that symptoms occurring for ≤1 mo are consistent with acute sinusitis. Chronic sinusitis is generally a consideration if symptoms have lasted >1 mo. Imaging studies with CT usually reveal mucosal thickening and ostial plugging if the sinusitis is chronic. *Recurrent sinusitis* is defined as >3 episodes/yr and should alert one to the possibility of immunodeficiency.

Causes

Pathophysiology
Acute sinusitis often develops when the sinus ostia become first obstructed, then infected. Local processes perpetuating this process include ostial narrowing secondary to mucosal inflammation after a viral infection or secondary to chronic changes from allergic disease. Immune deficiency and problems with the mucociliary transport, as well as predisposing anatomic factors, also lead to ostial narrowing. In the development of chronic sinusitis, however, other factors play a role; they include continued inflammation despite medical intervention, decreased O_2 delivery, microbial breakdown products, and continued inflammation influencing normal ciliary function, as well as organisms involved in the infection itself that may or may not be more pathogenic in nature.

Differential Diagnosis
Differential diagnosis is similar to allergic rhinitis (Table 3-1).
    INFECTIOUS ETIOLOGIES. Infectious etiologies are viral, bacterial, or fungal:

- **Viruses** are the most common cause of acute sinusitis and often invade before ensuing bacterial infection.
- The **most common bacterial etiologies** in acute sinusitis are *S. pneumoniae*, *H. influenzae*, and *Moraxella catarrhalis* (in children). *Staphylococcus aureus*, coagulase-negative *Staphylococcus*, and anaerobic bacteria are more commonly associated with chronic sinusitis. *Pseudomonas aeruginosa* frequently occurs in patients with cystic fibrosis.
- **Allergic fungal sinusitis** is rare. The hallmark feature is the presence of sinus opacification due to accumulation of "allergic mucin"—namely, thick, inspissated secretions heavily laden with eosinophils, Charcot-Leyden crystals, and fungal hyphae.

TABLE 3-1. DIFFERENTIAL DIAGNOSIS OF SINUSITIS

Upper respiratory viral infection

Rhinitis (allergic, nonallergic, vasomotor, occupational)

Hormonal rhinitis (hypothyroidism, pregnancy)

NARES

Aspirin sensitivity

Nasal polyposis

Drug-induced rhinitis (beta-blockers, ACE inhibitors, oral contraceptives, aspirin, NSAIDs)

Rhinitis medicamentosa (nasal decongestants, cocaine)

Allergic fungal sinusitis

Infectious fungal sinusitis

Anatomic variants

Tumors, foreign bodies

CSF rhinorrhea

- In the **immunocompromised** patient, **infectious fungal sinusitis:** *Aspergillus fumigatus* is the most common cause of fungal sinusitis and should always be considered in an immunocompromised patient. Other conditions predisposing to infectious fungal sinusitis include diabetes mellitus, leukemia, neutropenia, high-dose steroid therapy (as with connective tissue diseases), and immunosuppressive therapy. It is important to consider this problem, because infectious fungal sinusitis can rapidly become invasive (with local extension into the brain) or systemic, resulting in a poor prognosis.

ALLERGIC RHINITIS. Allergic rhinitis is an IgE-mediated inflammation of the nasal mucosa associated with watery rhinorrhea, allergic conjunctivitis, postnasal drainage, and sneezing that occurs in temporal relationship to allergen exposure.

NONALLERGIC RHINITIS EOSINOPHILIA SYNDROME. NARES is similar to allergic rhinitis, but there is no evidence of allergic disease by skin testing.

MEDICATIONS. Medications, such as aspirin, NSAIDS, beta-blockers, and ACE inhibitors, may cause rhinitis.

RHINITIS MEDICAMENTOSA. Repeated use of topical nasal decongestants may lead to rebound nasal congestion and hypertrophy of the nasal mucosa known as **rhinitis medicamentosa**.

VASOMOTOR RHINITIS. Vasomotor rhinitis is chronic nasal congestion secondary to excessive vasomotor activity. It has an unknown cause and is exacerbated by odors, temperature changes, and sunlight.

ANATOMIC OBSTRUCTION. Anatomic obstruction by foreign bodies (especially in children), nasal polyps, septal deviation, and tumors should always be considered.

Presentation

Predisposing Factors
Conditions that disrupt mucociliary clearance of secretions and promote ostial obstruction predispose patients to sinusitis. These include allergic rhinitis, nasal polyps, occupational rhinitis, and anatomic abnormalities, such as a foreign body. Sinusitis is less commonly a manifestation of systemic illnesses, such as immunodeficiency (including HIV, IgA, IgG, or IgG subclass deficiency), cystic fibrosis, immotile cilia syndrome, and Wegener's granulomatosis (Table 3-2).

History and Physical Exam
Patients often complain of purulent rhinorrhea, headache, nasal congestion, facial or dental pain or pressure, postnasal drip, and decrease or absence of olfaction (hyposmia or anosmia). Acute sinusitis symptoms within the first 7–10 days of illness almost always signify a viral rhinosinusitis and are recommended to be treated symptomatically rather than with antibiotics. Rhinosinusitis symptoms persisting beyond 7–10 days more commonly represent acute bacterial sinusitis.

Signs of sinusitis include a thick purulent discharge, mucosal erythema, tenderness to palpation over the sinuses, fetid breath, and mild periorbital edema. Marked periorbital edema, orbital pain or swelling, diplopia, ophthalmoplegia, and alterations of consciousness are **ominous signs** and necessitate emergency evaluation to exclude orbital cellulitis, cavernous vein thrombosis, meningitis, or brain abscess. One should also evaluate for any of the signs of allergic disease discussed earlier in this chapter (see Allergic Rhinitis). Clubbing of the nails may indicate the possibility of cystic fibrosis or Kartagener's syndrome. The presence of nasal polyposis suggests chronic sinusitis or, in children, cystic fibrosis.

Management

Diagnosis
The etiology of a patient's sinusitis may be apparent after a thorough history and physical exam. However, further evaluation is usually necessary.

IMAGING. The **Water's view** on plain film is useful for evaluating presence of maxillary sinusitis, while the **Caldwell view** is helpful for evaluating ethmoid and frontal

TABLE 3-2. PREDISPOSING FACTORS FOR SINUSITIS

Local

Upper respiratory infection

Rhinitis (allergic and nonallergic)

Anatomic variants

Hypertrophied adenoids

Nasal polyps, chronic mucosal thickening

Nasal or sinus tumors

Foreign bodies, cigarette smoke

Swimming and diving, barotrauma

Rhinitis medicamentosa, cocaine abuse

Nasal intubation

Periapical abscess in a protruding tooth

Systemic

Hypogammaglobulinemia

IgA deficiency

Panhypogammaglobulinemia

Specific antibody deficiency

IgG subclass deficiency

AIDS

Cystic fibrosis

Ciliary dysmotility syndromes

Kartagener's syndrome

Young's syndrome

Wegener's granulomatosis

---

sinuses. A four-view plain film **sinus series** is a helpful screening tool in the acute setting but is insensitive to ethmoid disease.

The **"limited" sinus CT scan** has become the most widely used radiographic study for diagnosis of sinusitis. It is obtained in the coronal projection with cuts through the frontal sinus, anterior ethmoid/maxillary sinuses, and posterior ethmoid and sphenoid sinuses. This scan allows for assessment of patency of the ostiomeatal unit, the critical confluence of drainage from the maxillary and anterior ethmoid sinuses.

MRI, while expensive, is useful for evaluating allergic or infectious fungal sinusitis and soft tissue extension. It is not good for evaluating mucosal thickening or bony deformities and, therefore, should not be used as an initial imaging method.

NASAL CYTOLOGY. Nasal cytology can be helpful but is rarely done. For this test, patients are asked to obtain a sample of their nasal discharge. The sample is then stained. Presence of eosinophils may indicate allergic rhinitis, NARES, aspirin sensitivity, or nasal polyps. Neutrophils are more indicative of infection.

LAB ANALYSIS. **Sweat chloride** testing should be performed if a child with nasal polyps presents with sinusitis. If **immunodeficiency** is suspected, quantitative immunoglobin levels should be obtained, and antibody production pre- and postimmunization with tetanus toxoid and pneumococcal polysaccharide vaccinations should be assessed.

BIOPSY. Biopsy is indicated if there is suspicion of a tumor or vasculitis. A biopsy may also be helpful to confirm the presence of invasive fungal infection.

CILIARY FUNCTION TESTING. Ciliary function testing is indicated in the setting of recurrent otitis, sinusitis, and pneumonia with bronchiectasis (Kartagener's syndrome). It is possible to do ciliary visual assessments, but a practical approach in the office setting is the saccharine test. This test involves placing a small amount of saccharine on the anterior portion of the inferior turbinate and timing when the patient begins to taste a sweet taste. A time to taste of >15–30 mins indicates a problem with cilia. Electron microscopy is the only way to document abnormal cilia structure.

RHINOSCOPY. The flexible fiberoptic rhinoscope can provide important information about presence or absence of purulent secretions, patency of sinus outflow tracts, nasal turbinate size, edema surrounding the eustachian tube orifices, hypertrophy of adenoidal tissue, and appearance of the sinus mucosa. Rhinoscopy is also an excellent tool for postop evaluation of patients for signs of infection, edema, polypoid changes or recurrence of nasal polyps. A summary of workup and management of the patient with chronic sinusitis is shown in Figs. 3-1 and 3-2.

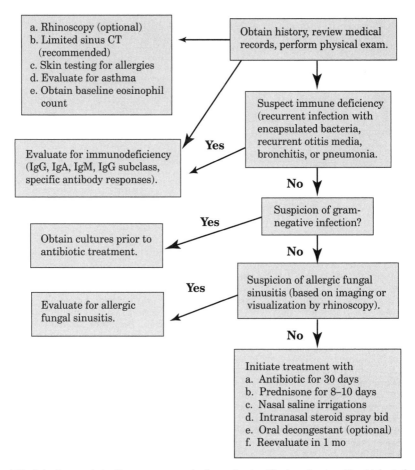

FIG. 3-1. Approach to the management of a patient with chronic sinusitis. [Adapted from Hamilos D. Chronic sinusitis. *J Allergy Clin Immunol* 2000;106(2):213–227.]

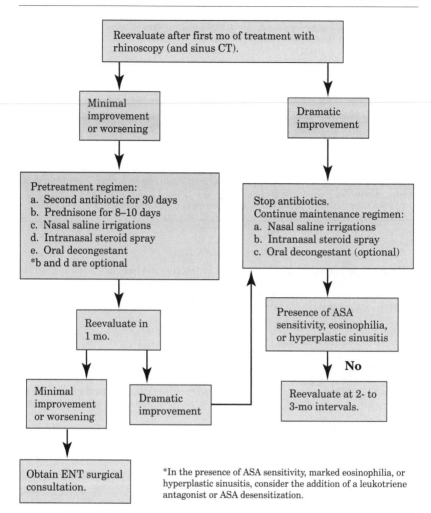

FIG. 3-2. Reevaluation of the patient after initial treatment of chronic sinusitis. [Adapted from Hamilos D. Chronic sinusitis. *J Allergy Clin Immunol* 2000;106(2):213–227.]

Treatment

ANTIBIOTICS. First-line treatments as recommended by consensus guidelines are amoxicillin (Amoxil, Biomox, Polymox, Trimox, Wymox) or trimethoprim-sulfamethoxazole (Bactrim, Septra) (TMP-SMX). Keep in mind that TMP-SMX frequently causes allergic reactions. In the case of a penicillin-allergic patient, other options include quinolones, cephalosporins, or macrolides. Acute sinusitis should be treated for ≥14 days, and patients should be instructed to fully complete the course of therapy. There is, however, increasing resistance to first-line therapies secondary to beta-lactamase production (e.g., *H. influenza, M. catarrhalis*) or, in the case of *S. pneumoniae*, alterations in penicillin-binding proteins. More than one-third of *H. influenza* strains, and virtually all *M. catarrhalis* strains, are penicillin resistant. Therefore, antibiotics with a beta-lactamase inhibitor should be considered, especially if the patient has not responded to first-line therapy within 1 wk or symptoms persist after therapy. In these cases, consider changing antibiotics to cover resistant organisms for another 7–10 days. In cases in which treatment has failed despite 3–4 wks of therapy, consider obtaining a bacterial sinus culture or a limited sinus CT before giving additional empiric therapy. If a patient has more than 3 episodes of sinusitis/year, consider evaluation for anatomic problems or immunodeficiency. Figs. 3-1 and 3-2 provide an algorithm for evaluation of a patient with chronic sinusitis.

INTRANASAL STEROIDS. Intranasal steroids are helpful in treatment of chronic sinusitis and, when combined with antibiotic therapy, may lessen the severity of symptoms of acute sinusitis.

DECONGESTANTS. Decongestants, such as inhaled phenylephrine, are potent vasoconstrictors that decrease swelling associated with mucosal inflammation. They are appropriately used for 3–5 days to alleviate symptoms but should be discontinued within this time to prevent rebound congestion and rhinitis medicamentosa. Oral decongestants are frequently used for symptomatic relief in acute and chronic sinusitis.

SALINE WASHES. Saline washes help in the setting of chronic sinusitis.

ORAL STEROIDS. Oral steroids are helpful in patients with chronic sinusitis to decrease inflammation and help restore normal mucociliary function (see Figs. 3-1 and 3-2).

REFERRAL. Indications for referral to an ENT surgeon are as follows:

- Evidence of anatomic defects by CT or physical exam, including foreign bodies, tumors, and nasal polyps that obstruct sinus drainage despite medical treatment.
- Persistent sinusitis despite aggressive medical management.
- Sinus condition requiring biopsy.
- Sinusitis complicated by extension into local structures, which includes evidence of brain abscess, cavernous sinus thrombosis, or erosion of the ethmoid or frontal sinuses.

KEY POINTS

- Nasal congestion, rhinorrhea, sneezing, and nasal itching are most commonly caused by allergic rhinitis, but **other causes of rhinitis need to be considered**.
- Seasonality of symptoms, specific **triggers**, positive **family history**, and **positive skin tests** are the hallmarks of allergic rhinitis.
- Skin tests for aeroallergans **are less expensive and more specific** than RAST in allergic rhinitis.
- **Environmental modification** and **intransal steroids** are the mainstays of treatment for allergic rhinitis.
- Symptoms of sinus infection **persisting more than 7–10 days** usually indicate bacterial sinusitis requiring **antibiotic therapy**.
- The **limited sinus CT** has become the most widely used radiographic study for the diagnosis of sinusitis.

SUGGESTED READING

Dykewicz MS, Fineman S, et al. Diagnosis and management of rhinitis: complete guidelines of the joint task force on practice parameters in allergy, asthma and immunology. *Ann Allergy Asthma Immunol* 1998;81(5):478–515.

Hamilos D. Chronic sinusitis. *J Allergy Clin Immunol* 2000;106(2):213–227.

Kay AB. Allergy and allergic diseases—second of two parts. *N Engl J Med* 2001;344(2): 109–113.

Middleton CE, Reed EF, Ellis NF, et al., eds. *Allergy: principles and practice*, 5th ed. St. Louis: Mosby, 1998.

Naclerio R, Solomon W. Rhinitis and inhalant allergens. *JAMA* 1997;278(22):1842–1848.

Slavin R. Nasal polyps and sinusitis. *JAMA* 1997;278(22):1849–1854.

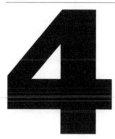

Asthma

Elizabeth C. Friedman

INTRODUCTION

Definition

Asthma is an inflammatory disorder of the lungs characterized by recurrent episodes of breathlessness, wheezing, coughing, and chest tightness, termed **exacerbations**, the severity of which can range from mild to life threatening. Asthma is also characterized by variable airflow obstruction that is reversible, either spontaneously or with therapy [1]. The majority of children who develop asthma do so on the basis of an underlying allergic diathesis. Adult-onset asthma's cause is either a continuum of allergic disease or based on other etiologies, such as occupational exposures.

Epidemiology

Asthma Epidemic

For reasons that are as yet unclear, asthma has been increasing in prevalence over the last 30 yrs. Worldwide and in the United States, the last several decades have seen an increase of approximately 5–7% per yr. There is a large variation in asthma prevalence throughout the world, with developed nations having the highest prevalence and Eastern Europe and developing countries having the lowest [2]. No clear evidence accounts for the epidemic and prevalence patterns; the increases are clearly too rapid to be explained by a change in genetic predisposition. A number of theories have been proposed.

HYGIENE HYPOTHESIS AND Th1/Th2 PARADIGM. At birth, T lymphocytes are naturally skewed toward a cytokine profile referred to as a *Th2*. Through development and challenge from infection, one's T cells normally develop a Th1 profile. The hygiene hypothesis suggests that the prevention of many childhood illnesses by vaccines and cleaner living conditions have suppressed this switch. In a group with a genetic predisposition to remain skewed toward a Th2 profile, the atopic or allergic phenotype develops [3].

POLLUTION. The increased incidence of asthma in the inner city suggests pollution as an environmental factor. However, although it has been shown to contribute to exacerbations, no causality has yet been determined [4].

ALTERED GI TRACT FLORA. Altered GI tract flora are thought to be secondary to increased antibiotic use in the first year of life [5].

Socioeconomic Factors

Several studies have demonstrated a higher prevalence, morbidity, and mortality in blacks vs whites in the United States. The highest mortality is seen in the poorest black inner-city neighborhoods [1]. Studies have also shown that mortality is related to severity rather than to excess ER use by this group [4].

Adult vs Pediatric Prevalence

In the United States, approximately 14 million people are affected; 4.8 million of these are children—roughly 5% of the population. Disease prevalence is greater among children and has increased the most in children <5 yrs, making it the most common chronic pediatric illness. Each year, there are 1.8 million ER visits and >460,000 hospitalizations [6].

Cost
In 1998, the National Heart, Lung, and Blood Institute (NHLBI) estimated that the annual costs of asthma were $11.3 billion/yr. This estimate includes $7.5 billion in direct medical expenses and $3.8 billion in indirect expenses, such as lost workdays for adults with asthma and lifetime earnings lost due to mortality from asthma [1].

Number of Deaths Annually
In addition to increased prevalence, a 25% increase in asthma-related deaths occurred in North America from 1960 to 1988, after which there has been a period of stabilization. In 1995, 5,637 people died from asthma. The 1997 figures show a decrease in the mortality rate for the first time since 1971; improved management is the likely explanation [7]. Asthma mortality rates are higher for women than men and for blacks than whites [8].

CAUSES

Pathophysiology

Inflammatory Condition
Denudation of airway epithelium, mucous plugging of segmental bronchi, collagen deposition beneath the basement membrane, edema of the submucosa, a predominantly eosinophilic infiltrate, and mucous cell metaplasia are among the histologic features of asthma. In addition to histamine, a host of inflammatory cytokines (e.g., IL-4, IL-13), chemokines (e.g., RANTES, eotaxin), cysteinyl leukotrienes (e.g., LTC_4, LTD_4), signal transduction-activation transcription (STAT) factors, and adhesion molecules are involved [3].

Hyperresponsiveness
Another central feature of asthma is bronchial hyperresponsiveness to nonspecific stimuli such as exercise or cold air and particularly viral URIs.

Etiology of Allergic Asthma
The majority of children with asthma are atopic with an additional susceptibility (not all patients with atopy have asthma). To assume that a particular allergen causes a direct inflammatory reaction in the lungs is an oversimplification, because most inhaled allergens are filtered in the nose and upper airway before reaching the small airways. Several candidate genes have been proposed (Table 4-1), although research in this area is difficult because of the disease's heterogeneity. For example, many children with asthma "outgrow" the disease, whereas other individuals develop progressive symptoms and chronic airway remodeling.

Differential Diagnosis (or "All That Wheezes Is Not Asthma")
- COPD
- CHF
- Postviral RAD
- Mechanical airway obstruction, including tracheal stenosis, tracheomalacia, neoplasm or inflammatory mass, foreign body
- Extrathoracic obstruction, including vocal cord dysfunction
- Pulmonary embolism
- Gastroesophageal reflux
- Chronic eosinophilic pneumonia
- Churg-Strauss syndrome

TABLE 4-1. LINKAGES WITH ALLERGY AND ASTHMA CHROMOSOME CANDIDATE GENES OR PRODUCTS

1p	IL-12 receptor
2p	IL-1, cytotoxic T lymphocyte–associated antigen 4, CD28
3p24	B-cell lymphoma-6 (STAT-6 binding inhibition)
	Chemokine cell receptor 4
5q23-35	IL-3, IL-4, IL-5, IL-9, IL-13, GM-CSF
	LTC_{4S}
	Macrophage colony-stimulating factor receptor
	$Beta_2$-adrenergic receptor
	Glucocorticosteroid receptor
	TIM1, TIM3
6p21-23	MHC
	TNFs
	Transporters involved in antigen processing and presentation (TAP1 and TAP3)
	Large multicatalytic proteolytic particles
7q11-14	T-cell receptor g chain, IL-6
11q13	High-affinity IgE receptor (FcεRI) beta chain
	Clara cell protein 16
	Fibroblast growth factor 3
12q14-24	IFN-gamma
	Stem cell factor
	Nitric oxide synthetase (constitutive)
	Beta subunit of nuclear factor Y (transcription factor for HLA gene)
	Insulinlike growth factor
	Leukotriene A_4 hydrolase
	STAT-6 (IL-4 STAT)
13q21-24	Cysteinyl leukotriene 2 receptor
14q11-13	T-cell receptor alpha and delta chains
	Nuclear factor kappaB inhibitor
16p11-12	IL-4 receptor
17p12-17	CC chemokine cluster
19q13CD22	Transforming growth factor $beta_1$
20p13	ADAM-33

Natural History

A large, prospective study of children in Tucson, Arizona, demonstrated several important features about **childhood asthma**:

- Wheezing seen only in the first year of life is dependent on airway size and does not predict future asthma.

- Children who continue to wheeze beyond age 2 are at risk for developing asthma.
- Some children who are at risk for asthma will not develop symptoms until after age 2.
- Independent risk factors for asthma include maternal smoking and a maternal history of asthma [9].

Other data suggest that exposure of young children to older children at home or to other children at day care protects against the development of asthma and frequent wheezing later in childhood [10].

Another study suggests that **respiratory syncytial virus** is an independent risk factor for wheezing in children until age 11 but not after age 13 [11].

PRESENTATION

General Features

- The hallmark of asthma is reversibility.
- Patients exhibit hypersensitivity to nonspecific triggers and/or viral respiratory infections.
- **Nocturnal awakenings** with coughing or wheezing may be the presenting symptom, **especially in children**. Nocturnal symptoms in a patient who has previously had only daytime symptoms represent disease progression. Circadian fluctuations in cortisol alone do not explain nocturnal symptoms. Intense dust exposure in bedding, waning of daytime medications, postural changes, and sleep-related changes in mucociliary clearance may play a role [12].
- **Exercise-induced bronchospasm** may also be the presenting symptom. Consider asthma if a child cannot keep up with peers during athletic activity secondary to coughing or wheezing.

Features of Acute Exacerbations

Some or all of these may be present:

- **Shortness of breath**, particularly with exertion.
- **Chest tightness or pain**.
- **Wheezing** may be audible to the patient but often is not.
- **Cough**: often productive secondary to inspissated secretions without necessarily being related to an infectious cause. Some patients rarely wheeze but **cough** instead, **especially children**. This is an important feature that should not be missed, because patients with **cough variant asthma** generally respond well to therapy but often go undiagnosed. (Note: marked dyspnea and agitation in a patient who can speak in full sentences should cause one to consider vocal cord dysfunction.)

Physical Exam

Between exacerbations, the exam may be completely normal!

Vital Signs
Often normal, even in an acute exacerbation. One may see elevated heart and respiratory rates.

General Appearance
Does the patient appear dyspneic? Can the patient speak in full sentences? The patient in respiratory distress may become agitated. A patient who has become lethargic is in danger of respiratory failure.

HEENT Exam
The HEENT exam may show signs of allergic disease or an upper respiratory tract infection. Note accessory muscle use in the neck. This is more common in children; in

adults, it suggests the diagnosis of COPD. Stridor or wheezing best heard in the neck suggests an alternative diagnosis, such as vocal cord dysfunction or upper airway obstruction.

Lung Exam
High-pitched end expiratory wheeze is most typical. One may hear cough with forced expiratory maneuvers. In severe asthma, one may not hear a wheeze at all. **Beware the patient who has stopped wheezing, since if accompanied by lethargy, respiratory failure may be imminent.** Rhonchi or focal findings suggest a pulmonary infection that may have triggered the exacerbation, although, if unaccompanied by fever or other signs of infection, they may represent the tenacious secretions commonly seen in asthmatics. Respiratory muscle alternans is the paradoxic movement of the diaphragm with alternating abdominal and ribcage breathing. It represents a patient in extremis and is more commonly seen in children.

Rest of Exam
Note intercostal retractions, particularly in children. Note signs of Cushing's syndrome secondary to exogenous oral steroid use. Also note signs and symptoms of comorbidities or confounding conditions.

MANAGEMENT

Lab Analysis

General Labs
Lab results are generally normal. One may see an elevated WBC count in settings of infection or oral steroid use (note that the leukocytosis is a neutrophilia in steroid use; more immature forms suggest an infection). Routine chemistries are usually normal. Pulsus paradoxus may be present (see Fig. 4-1).

Peak Expiratory Flow
The "peak flow" measurement does not itself diagnose asthma; a full set of lung functions is necessary. However, it is probably the best way to monitor a patient's response to therapy during an exacerbation and as an outpatient. In the acute setting, it is helpful to check peak flows before and after bronchodilator use and keep a chart of these values at the patient's bedside during a hospital stay or ER visit.

Pulmonary Function Tests
Pulmonary function tests reveal an obstructive pattern with diminished expiratory flow rate (see Chap. 7, Pulmonary Function Tests). The flow volume loop can aid in the diagnosis of vocal cord dysfunction, but only when the patient is symptomatic.

Bronchoprovocation Tests
The gold standard for diagnosis of asthma is the methacholine challenge.

Chest X-Ray
An initial chest x-ray (CXR) of a pediatric patient who is wheezing for the first time is necessary to rule out aspiration of a foreign body. It should also be obtained on any patient requiring admission. This exam is rarely necessary in the outpatient setting for an established asthmatic. Even in a patient with concomitant COPD, CXR will not delineate how much of the disease is related to asthma, since many of the findings are the same: hyperinflation (flattening of the diaphragms) and mucous plugging (linear atelectasis). However, there are several situations in which CXR might be useful, such as patients who present with new-onset wheezing, have other comorbidities (e.g., congestive heart failure, COPD, or pneumonia), or have focal findings on exam. One should also obtain a CXR when suspicion of a pneumothorax or pneumomediastinum is present.

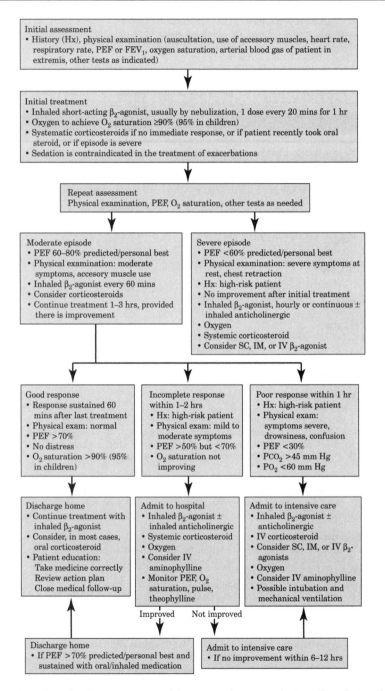

FIG. 4-1. Algorithm for management of the acute asthma exacerbation. (From Lemanske RF Jr, Busse WW. Asthma. *JAMA* 1997;278:1855–1873, with permission.)

Aeroallergen Skin Tests and Environmental History

As stated in the section Etiology of Allergic Asthma, most patients develop asthma on the basis of allergic disease. Thus, no initial outpatient evaluation would be complete without a detailed environmental history. This history includes details about the home/work/school environment, animal exposure, smoking history or passive smoke exposure, whether the patient has a seasonal or perennial profile of symptoms, and any family history of atopy. Skin testing is often useful to guide therapy and allergen avoidance and thus is recommended in any evaluation of new-onset asthma.

Blood Gas

Most important to recognize is the patient in danger of respiratory failure. Few patients presenting for a simple asthma exacerbation require a blood gas. However, it is **warranted if the patient is in status asthmaticus and requires ICU admission**. It may also be useful when the patient has other comorbidities, particularly COPD or pneumonia. Most patients will have an accompanying **respiratory alkalosis** from hyperventilation as the patient works to increase minute ventilation. **Caution: A patient whose CO_2 is normal or above normal during a severe exacerbation is in danger of respiratory failure**. This "normal" value represents a patient who can no longer maintain a high minute ventilation and has begun to tire out. **This patient requires hospital admission** and immediate aggressive intervention, such as endotracheal intubation or another mode of assisted ventilation [13].

Asthma Complications

Status Asthmaticus

Status asthmaticus is defined as a severe exacerbation that fails to respond rapidly to sympathomimetic agents. Patients at risk for status are those who are on oral steroids, who smoke, who have previously been intubated, who have been admitted to an ICU within the last year, and who frequently or recently visited the ER [14]. Although deaths from asthma are infrequent, mortality is on the increase. Patients are more likely to die from their asthma if they have psychiatric illness (underdiagnosed in severe asthmatics), use bronchodilators excessively or do not use **inhaled corticosteroids (ICS),** and use the ER as their primary means of accessing the healthcare system [15].

Chronic Airway Remodeling

Although one may assume that patients with severe persistent asthma are at risk for persistent obstruction, no criteria or distinguishing features have been defined regarding this subset of patients. In fact, it is not always the most symptomatic patient whose disease will progress. Although inhaled steroids have become the mainstay of treatment, it is unclear whether they are disease-modifying drugs. However, it is clear that even low doses of ICS decrease asthma mortality [16].

Allergic Bronchopulmonary Aspergillosis

Allergic bronchopulmonary aspergillosis (ABPA) is a complication of asthma and cystic fibrosis originally described by Hinson in 1952. To date, its diagnosis, classification, and treatment remain controversial.

Aspergillus fumigatus is a common environmental mold that, in the immunocompromised host, can cause invasive disease. It is also a common allergen to which many atopic patients are sensitized that contributes to both asthma and allergic rhinitis.

ABPA represents colonization with *Aspergillus* rather than tissue invasion. In a small subset of patients who likely have a genetic susceptibility, asthma progresses to intractable disease and, often, oral corticosteroid (OCS)–dependent disease [24]. The diagnosis is made by meeting several criteria (Table 4-2), and the disease is classified into stages (Table 4-3). It should be noted that no single test diagnoses ABPA, and diagnosis can be difficult in a patient on steroids or in remission because of the lack of eosinophilia.

TABLE 4-2. DIAGNOSTIC CRITERIA FOR ALLERGIC BRONCHOPULMONARY ASPERGILLOSIS

Clinical or lab feature	Essential for diagnosis?
Asthma	Yes
Chest roentgenographic infiltrate	No
Immediate cutaneous reactivity to *Aspergillus*	Yes
Elevated total IgE[a]	Yes, >1,000 ng/mL
Precipitating antibodies to Af[a]	Yes
Peripheral blood eosinophilia[a]	No
Elevated serum IgE-Af and IgG-Af	Yes
Central bronchiectasis[b]	No

[a]May be diminished or absent in a patient on oral steroid therapy.
[b]In the absence of cystic fibrosis, the *sine qua non* of allergic bronchopulmonary aspergillosis.
From Greenberger PA, Patterson R. Diagnosis and management of allergic bronchopulmonary aspergillosis. *Ann Allergy* 1986;56:444–452, with permission.

Concerns in the Asthmatic Patient Hospitalized for Other Reasons
Patients with asthma who are hospitalized for other reasons should continue appropriate outpatient medications unless contraindicated. **ICS are often neglected on admission orders either by the housestaff or by the patient who fails to list them.** It is not appropriate to place patients on scheduled doses of bronchodilators in place of their regular therapy. It is reasonable to check a **theophylline (Bronkodyl, Elixophyllin, Slo-bid, Slo-Phyllin, Theo-24) level** if the patient is on theophylline, because it has a narrow therapeutic window and the ability to interact with numerous other medications. Patients who have been on oral steroids for >3 wks in the previous year should be monitored for signs of adrenal insufficiency and given **stress dose steroids** as needed (usually 100 mg hydrocortisone q8h). Patients requiring intubation may have issues related to hyperinflation and are at risk for barotrauma. For specific ventilator management, see the section Features of Ventilator Management.

Vocal Cord Dysfunction
Vocal cord dysfunction consists of voluntary or involuntary adduction of the true or false vocal cords. This disorder is far more prevalent than realized by most clinicians. It has been suggested that up to **40% of asthmatics** exhibit this behavior. Patients often report instantaneous onset of their asthma symptoms; they display a weak voice when symptomatic and complain of a choking sensation. **Wheezing is heard in the larynx**, and the **flow volume loop** of a pulmonary function test shows a characteristic **flat inspiratory curve**. However, **diagnosis is made definitively by rhinoscopy**.

TABLE 4-3. STAGING OF ALLERGIC BRONCHOPULMONARY ASPERGILLOSIS

Stage I	Acute
Stage II	Remission
Stage III	Exacerbation
Stage IV	Corticosteroid-dependent asthma
Stage V	Fibrotic

From Greenberger PA, Patterson R. Diagnosis and management of allergic bronchopulmonary aspergillosis. *Ann Allergy* 1986;56:444–452, with permission.

Treatment consists of speech therapy. Early intervention is key, because many patients end up on prolonged courses of oral steroids for what is believed to be intractable asthma. Many patients also benefit from psychiatric treatment, as at least half have an underlying depression, conversion disorder, or histrionic personality disorder, or, at the very least, maladaptive coping skills.

Status Asthmaticus

In the words of Dr. Thomas Petty, "the best treatment of status asthmaticus is to treat it 3 days before it occurs." Despite optimal outpatient care, patients occasionally present with a life-threatening exacerbation.

SUMMARY OF WHEN TO ACT QUICKLY

- Tachycardia (>120 bpm)
- Tachypnea (>30 breaths/min)
- Diaphoresis
- Inability to lie supine
- Pulsus paradox >10 mm Hg

Important note: The absence of these signs does not rule out respiratory failure; **physical exam cannot be relied on exclusively to estimate the severity of airway obstruction**. Wheezing may diminish as lung volumes decrease; therefore, a patient with severe obstruction may have minimal wheezing on exam.

IMPENDING RESPIRATORY FAILURE. The following represent impending respiratory failure:

- Respiratory muscle alternans
- Depressed mental status
- Elevated CO_2 on arterial blood gas

FEATURES OF VENTILATOR MANAGEMENT. The goal of ventilator management is adequate oxygenation with the least risk for barotrauma. Ventilated patients in status have a much higher ventilation/perfusion mismatch and a higher ventilatory requirement than do patients with COPD; thus, they are particularly at risk for barotrauma.

- **Controlled hypoventilation** and **permissive hypercapnia:** a bicarb drip is only necessary for patients with pH <7.2.
- **Low tidal volumes:** 6 cc/kg of ideal body weight.
- **Low respiratory rate:** to allow for long expiratory phase.
- Peak pressure <35.
- Plateau pressure <30.
- Inspiratory flow <60 L/min.
- Low positive end expiratory pressure.
- **Sedation:** Aggressive sedation is necessary for a patient in status to synchronize with the ventilator. **Paralysis should be used with caution:** Patients on steroids are at increased risk of myopathy. Benzodiazepines are the sedative of choice; avoid opiates that are nonspecific mast cell degranulators, because in some patients they can make bronchospasm worse [17].
- **Alternative therapies:** Debate continues regarding the use of theophylline in status. Anticholinergics appear to add little to inhaled beta-agonists. **Routine use of magnesium sulfate or antibiotics in status is not recommended**.

Asthma during Pregnancy

The response of asthma to pregnancy is variable. Roughly one-third of women improve during pregnancy, one-third do not change, and one-third deteriorate. There has been concern about the use of systemic steroids and risk to the fetus. However, it has also been recognized that the risk to the fetus from hypoxia is far worse and may have been a confounding factor in some of these studies. Thus, the treatment algorithm generally remains the same as in the nonpregnant patient, with the caveat that unnecessary medications should not be given in the first trimester.

Treatment

An algorithm for management of acute exacerbations from guidelines published by the NHLBI is reproduced in Fig. 4-1 [1]. The NHLBI's stepwise treatment algorithm is covered in Table 4-4 [1].

Avoidance of Allergens/Triggers and Asthma Action Plan

One study shows a 70% reduction in the risk of death for patients with a written asthma management or "action" plan [19]. This plan should include written instructions for monitoring and responding to symptoms, as well as instructions in the use of medication delivery devices and a peak flow meter. Patients should also be aware of triggers/allergens and understand how to avoid them. They should be given information on instituting appropriate environmental controls in the home. It is also important to treat comorbid conditions, such as allergic rhinitis and chronic sinusitis, as these can contribute to increased severity of asthma [21].

Beta-Adrenergic Agents: Short Acting

Short-acting beta-adrenergic agents [albuterol (Proventil, Ventolin)] are the most potent and rapidly acting bronchodilators. Only patients with mild intermittent symptoms should use this class of medication as monotherapy. These drugs are referred to as "rescue" medications, indicating their use as symptom-controlling agents. They are also effective for premedicating exercise or a known allergen exposure (e.g., animals). This class can be administered by metered-dose inhaler, or nebulizer, or orally (liquid suspension). **The inhaled forms are recommended**, even in pediatric use, since side effects of tremor, tachycardia, and anxiety are minimized with proper inhaler technique using a spacer or with nebulized solution. **Increasing use of beta-agonists or use of >1 canister in 1 mo indicates inadequate asthma control and the need for initiation or intensification of antiinflammatory therapy.** Excessive use of short-acting beta-adrenergic agents may down-regulate the $beta_2$ receptor, causing increased airway hyperresponsiveness.

Inhaled Corticosteroids

ICS are the **mainstay of pharmacotherapy**. Mechanisms are antiinflammatory: blocking of late-phase reaction to allergens, reduction of airway hyperresponsiveness, inhibition of cytokine production, and reversal of $beta_2$-receptor down-regulation.

Patients are started on the dose needed to gain control of symptoms and are titrated down to the lowest dose needed to maintain control.

ICS are not "rescue" medicines. **The onset of action is several days**, with maximal effect in 2–3 wks. ICS can be stepped up during a mild exacerbation before using oral steroids (Table 4-4).

LOCAL SIDE EFFECTS. Local side effects are dysphonia, throat irritation, and oral candidiasis. These occurrences are not common, and patients can avoid thrush by rinsing their mouths after inhaler use.

SYSTEMIC EFFECTS. ICS are rapidly metabolized by the liver (first-pass effect) and have little systemic effect in adults. Patients who are transitioning from >3 wks of oral steroids are at risk for adrenal insufficiency.

There has been concern regarding bone growth in children. *Large, prospective studies have shown that children with asthma on ICS have a slightly delayed growth velocity compared to the placebo group. However, this delay is transient.* There is no question that uncontrolled asthma has detrimental effects on growth and development [18].

Oral Corticosteroids

OCS are the most potent antiinflammatory agents available to treat asthma. Their side effects are well known, ranging from adrenal insufficiency to Cushing's syndrome to avascular necrosis to glucose intolerance. Mood-altering effects can be quite pronounced, especially in the very young and old, ranging from hyperactivity to overt psychosis. Many patients are aware of these effects and resist taking the medication or giving it to their children, even in the setting of a severe exacerbation. Clinicians should explain to patients that only long-term use is a risk factor for most side effects

TABLE 4-4. STEPWISE APPROACH FOR MANAGING ASTHMA

	Long-term control	Quick relief	Education
Step 4: severe, persistent	Daily medications: **antiinflammatory: inhaled corticosteroid (high dose)** AND **Long-acting bronchodilator:** either **long-acting inhaled beta$_2$-agonist**, sustained release theophylline, or long-acting beta$_2$-agonist tablets AND Corticosteroid tablets or syrup long term (make repeat attempts to reduce systemic steroids and maintain control with high-dose inhaled steroids).	Short-acting bronchodilator: **inhaled beta$_2$-agonists** as needed for symptoms. Intensity of treatment depends on severity of exacerbation. Use of short-acting inhaled beta$_2$-agonists on a daily basis or increasing use indicates the need for additional long-term control therapy.	Steps 2 and 3 actions plus: Refer to individual education/counseling.
Step 3: moderate, persistent	Daily medication: Either **antiinflammatory: inhaled corticosteroid (medium dose)** OR Inhaled corticosteroid (low-medium dose) and add a long-acting bronchodilator, especially for nighttime symptoms; either **long-acting inhaled beta$_2$-agonist**, sustained-release theophylline, or long-acting beta$_2$-agonist tablets. If needed, antiinflammatory; **inhaled corticosteroids (medium-high dose)** AND **Long-acting bronchodilator**, especially for nighttime symptoms; either **long-acting inhaled beta$_2$-agonist**, sustained-release theophylline, or long-acting beta$_2$-agonist tablets. Inhaled beta$_2$-agonists as needed for symptoms.	Short-acting bronchodilator: **inhaled beta$_2$-agonists** as needed for symptoms. Intensity of treatment will depend on severity of exacerbation. Use of short-acting inhaled beta$_2$-agonists on a daily basis or increasing use indicates the need for additional long-term control therapy.	Step 1 actions plus: Teach self-monitoring. Refer to group education if available. Review and update self-management plan.
Step 2: mild, persistent	One daily medication: **antiinflammatory:** either **inhaled corticosteroid** (low doses) or **cromolyn or nedocromil** (children usually begin with a trial of cromolyn or nedocromil).	Short-acting bronchodilator: **inhaled beta$_2$-agonists** as needed for symptoms. Intensity of treatment will depend on severity of exacerbation.	Step 1 actions plus: Teach self-monitoring.

(continued)

TABLE 4-4. CONTINUED

	Long-term control	Quick relief	Education
	Sustained-release theophylline to serum concentration of 5–15 µg/mL is an alternative, but not preferred, therapy. Zafirlukast or zileuton may also be considered for patients ≥ 12 yrs of age, although their position in therapy is not fully established.	Use of short-acting inhaled beta$_2$-agonists on a daily basis or increasing use indicates the need for additional long-term control therapy.	Refer to group education if available. Review and update self-management plan.
Step 1: mild, intermittent	No daily medication needed.	Short-acting bronchodilator: inhaled beta$_2$-agonists as needed for symptoms. Intensity of treatment will depend on severity of exacerbation; see component 3-Managing Exacerbations. Use of short-acting inhaled beta$_2$-agonists more than 2×/wk may indicate the need to initiate long-term control therapy.	Teach basic facts about asthma. Teach inhaler/spacer/holding chamber technique. Discuss roles of medications. Develop self-management plan. Develop action plan for when and how to take rescue actions, especially for patients with a history of severe exacerbations. Discuss appropriate environmental control measures to avoid exposure to known allergens and irritants.

Step down: review treatment every 1–6 mos; a gradual stepwise reduction in treatment may be possible.

Step up: if control is not maintained, consider step up. First, review patient medication technique, adherence, and environmental control (avoidance of allergens or other factors that contribute to asthma severity).

Note: Preferred treatments are in bold.
The stepwise approach presents general guidelines to assist clinical decision making; it is not intended to be a specific prescription. Asthma is highly variable; clinicians should tailor specific medication plans to the needs and circumstances of individual patients.
Gain control as quickly as possible; then decrease treatment to the least medication necessary to maintain control. Gaining control may be accomplished by either starting treatment at the step most appropriate to the initial severity of the condition or starting at a higher level of therapy (e.g., a course of systemic corticosteroids or higher dose of inhaled corticosteroids).
A rescue course of systemic corticosteroids may be needed at any time and at any step.
Some patients with intermittent asthma experience severe and life-threatening exacerbations separated by long periods of normal lung function and no symptoms. This may be especially common with exacerbations provoked by respiratory infections. A short course of systemic corticosteroids is recommended.
At each step, patients should control their environment to avoid or control factors that make their asthma worse (e.g., allergens, irritants); this requires specific diagnosis and education.
Referral to an asthma specialist for consultation or co-management is *recommended* if there are difficulties achieving or maintaining control of asthma or if the patient requires step 4 care. Referral may be *considered* if the patient requires step 3 care.

and that **rapid control of an exacerbation and compliance with other medications afterward is the best strategy to avoid OCS use in the future.**

Tapering of OCS to avoid adrenal insufficiency is only necessary when a patient has taken them for >3 wks.

A patient is a candidate for an OCS burst during an asthma exacerbation if the symptoms are particularly severe or the patient requires more than a reasonable amount of rescue medication (see Fig. 4-1). **Any patient requiring hospitalization should be placed on parenteral or oral steroids.** Most clinicians give excessive doses of highly potent steroids in the initial phase of an exacerbation. See Fig. 4-1 for dosing recommendations.

Beta-Adrenergic Agents: Long Acting

Unlike short-acting bronchodilators, these medications [salmeterol (Serevent), formoterol (Foradil)] are not recommended in the acute setting. In fact, patients should be cautioned not to exceed the normal doses because of side effects (same as short-acting agents). Recent trials have determined that these long-acting agents have a synergistic effect with ICS, allowing for a smaller dose of each medication to control symptoms. Long-acting beta-agonists are especially helpful for controlling nocturnal symptoms [22,23].

Antileukotriene Drugs

Use of antileukotriene drugs [montelukast (Sinqulair) and zafirlukast (Accolate)] is a recent development in the asthma armamentarium, and, as such, their exact role remains to be fully determined. The antileukotriene drugs are more effective than placebo but less effective than ICS at improving peak expiratory flow rates, reducing $beta_2$-adrenergic use and increasing symptom-free days. They are particularly useful in several instances: **aspirin intolerance, exercise-induced symptoms, and problems using an inhaler** [20].

Allergen Immunotherapy

Patients with persistent symptoms despite efforts at allergen/trigger avoidance and pharmacotherapy may be candidates for immunotherapy (see Chap. 21, Allergen Immunotherapy). Its efficacy for asthmatics with pollen allergy has been established; other allergens have not been as well studied, but one would presume a similar benefit.

Nedocromil/Cromolyn Sodium

Nedocromil (Tilade) and cromolyn sodium (Intal, Intal Inhaler) are antiinflammatory medications effective in adult and pediatric patients. They are not as effective as inhaled steroids but should be considered in any patient with mild asthma for whom inhaled steroids cannot be used.

Theophylline

Theophylline (Uniphyl) is a methylxanthine in PO or IV form that acts as a bronchodilator. We have many years of experience with this medication; over the years, it has fallen in and out of favor. It is currently not a first-line agent in any circumstance for several reasons:

- Its onset of action is slower than that of beta-agonists.
- It has a very narrow therapeutic window, and toxicity is common.
- Its use is often limited by side effects (particularly GI), even at therapeutic levels.
- The number of interactions with medications and physiologic states (fever, diet) is legion.

Despite these limitations, it is an effective medication and has a role as adjunct therapy in the carefully monitored patient for both the acute and outpatient settings.

When to Use Antibiotics

It is widely recognized that one of the most common triggers for an asthma exacerbation is the viral upper respiratory tract infection, yet most patients who require oral steroids for a severe exacerbation inevitably end up on broad-spectrum antibiotics as well. That said, any patients hospitalized for their asthma who have concomitant respiratory tract infections deserve a course of a well-chosen antimicrobial agent. In the outpatient setting, it is often reasonable to treat the asthma by increasing the patient's inhaled steroid or using oral prednisone (Deltasone, Liquid Pred, Meticorten, Orasone, Prednicen-M, Sterapred, Sterapred DS). A viral infection can be treated symptomatically, but the patient must be carefully monitored; those not responding to the above measures should be considered for antimicrobial therapy.

KEY POINTS

- Only mild, intermittent asthma qualifies for monotherapy.
- Asthma is best treated by using enough medication to gain control of symptoms, then titrating down to the lowest doses needed to maintain control.
- The best time to treat "status asthmaticus" (or any exacerbation) is 3 days before it happens.

REFERENCES

1. National Heart, Lung, and Blood Institute. *Executive summary: guidelines for the diagnosis and management of asthma.* Bethesda, MD: U.S. Department of Health and Human Services, 1991. NIH publication 91-3042.
2. Beasley R, Keil V, vonMutius E, Pearce N. ISAAC Steering Committee: Worldwide variation in prevalence of symptoms of asthma, allergic rhinoconjunctivitis, and atopic eczema: ISAAC. *Lancet* 1998;351:1225–1232.
3. Busse WW, Lemanske RF. Advances in immunology: asthma. *N Engl J Med* 2001;344(5):350–362.
4. Hartert TV, Peebles RS. Epidemiology of asthma: the year in review. *Curr Opin Pulm Med* 2000;(1):4–9.
5. Mattes J, Karmaus W. The use of antibiotics in the first year of life and development of asthma: which comes first? *Clin Exp Allergy* 1999;29:729–732.
6. Mannino DM, Homa DM, Pertowski CA, et al. Surveillance for asthma—United States, 1960–1995. *MMWR Morb Mortal Wkly Rep* 1998;477(No. SS-1):1–27.
7. Sly RM. Decreases in asthma mortality in the United States. *Ann Allergy Asthma Immunol* 2000;85:121–127.
8. National Heart, Lung, and Blood Institute. Data fact sheet: asthma statistics 1999.
9. Martinez FD, Wright AL, Taussig LM, et al. Asthma and wheezing in the first six years of life. *N Engl J Med* 1995;332(3):133–138.
10. Ball TM, Castro-Rodriguez JA, Griffith KA, et al. Siblings, day-care attendance, and the risk of asthma and wheezing during childhood. *N Engl J Med* 2000;343(8):538–543.
11. Stein RT, Sherrill D, Morgan WJ, et al. Respiratory syncytial virus in early life and risk of wheeze and allergy by age 13 years. *Lancet* 1999;354:541–545.
12. Middleton E, Reed CE, Ellis EF, eds. *Allergy: principles and practice,* 5th ed. St. Louis: Mosby, 1998.
13. Madison JM, Irwin RS. Status asthmaticus. In: Rippe JM, et al., eds. *Intensive care medicine,* 3rd ed. Boston: Little, Brown, 1996;605–618.
14. Turner MO, Noertjojo K, Vedal S, et al. Risk factors for near-fatal asthma: a case control study in hospitalized patients with asthma. *Am J Respir Crit Care Med* 1998;157:1804–1809.
15. Corn B, Hamrung G, Ellis A, et al. Patterns of asthma death and near-death in an inner-city tertiary care teaching hospital. *J Asthma* 1995;32(6):405–412.
16. Suissa S, Ernst P. Inhaled corticosteroids: impact on asthma morbidity and mortality. *J Allergy Clin Immunol* 2001;107(6):937–944.
17. Corbridge TC, Hall JB. The assessment and management of adults with status asthmaticus. *Am J Respir Crit Care Med* 1995;151(5):1296–1316.
18. Szefler S, Weiss S, Tonascia J. Long term effects of budesonide or nedocromil in children with asthma: the Childhood Asthma Management Program (CAMP) Research Group. *N Engl J Med* 2000;343(15):1054–1063.

19. Abramson MJ, Bailey MJ, Couper FJ. Are asthma medications and management related to deaths from asthma? *Am J Respir Crit Care Med* 2001;163(1):8–12.
20. Smith LJ. Comparative efficacy of inhaled corticosteroids and antileukotriene drugs in asthma. *BioDrugs* 2001;15(4):239–249.
21. Simons FER. Allergic rhinobronchitis: the asthma–allergic rhinitis link. *J Allergy Clin Immunol* 1999;104:534–540.
22. Pauwels RA, Lofdahl CG, et al. Effect of inhaled formoterol and budesonide on exacerbations of asthma. *N Engl J Med* 1997;337:1405–1411.
23. Condemi JJ, Goldstein S, Kalberg C, et al. The addition of salmeterol to fluticasone propionate in patients with persistent asthma. *Ann Allergy Asthma Immunol* 1999;82:383–389.
24. Chauhan B, Santiago L, Hutcheson PS, et al. Evidence for the involvement of two different MHC class II regions in susceptibility or protection in allergic bronchopulmonary aspergillosis. *J Allergy Clin Immunol* 2000;106:723–729.

Occupational Asthma

Alpa L. Jani

INTRODUCTION

Definition
Occupational asthma (OA) is defined as variable airflow limitation and/or bronchial hyperresponsiveness caused by exposures in, not outside, the workplace [1]. Within this definition, some authors may include asthma that is preexistent but made worse by exposure to the workplace, termed *work-aggravated asthma* [2].

Epidemiology
Defining the prevalence of OA is difficult, given the lack of prospective data across different industries and given recent advances in industrial safety. However, one study estimates that OA represents 2–6% of all adult asthma cases [3]. OA risk is best defined by industry because prevalence rates may vary, from 7–9% of bakers [4] to 25% in a group of platinum refinery workers [4].

Classification
OA is typically classified into OA with latency, the most common form, or OA without latency.

OA with Latency
OA with latency describes asthma that begins with exposure to a known sensitizer and is then followed by a period of latency (months to years) between first exposure and onset of symptoms. This type of OA is typically immunologically mediated and occurs in response to a high-molecular-weight (HMW) (>5 kd) sensitizer or in response to a haptenated low-molecular-weight (LMW) (<5 kd) chemical. Only a small percentage of workers will have symptoms when reexposed to low amounts of the sensitizer [5].

OA without Latency
Also termed *reactive airways dysfunction syndrome* (RADS) or *irritant-induced asthma*, OA without latency presents with the acute onset of asthma symptoms immediately after exposure to large amounts or high concentrations of vapors, gases, fumes, dust, or smoke. Such exposure typically occurs in the setting of a chemical spill or accident on the job. The symptoms usually drive the worker to seek emergency medical attention. In most cases, workers eventually recover completely, but some develop persistent symptoms of bronchial hyperreactivity. More recently, some authors have extended this condition's clinical spectrum to include those with bronchial reactivity resulting from recurrent low-dose exposures. However, this idea is controversial, with other authors proposing that these cases of "low-level RADS" may simply be cases of aggravated preexisting asthma [6].

CAUSES

Pathophysiology

More than 250 agents have been named as possible causes of occupational asthma [2]. These are divided into **HMW agents**, usually proteins >5 kd, and **LMW chemicals** that are <5 kd, and they can be further organized by their pathogenic mechanisms, as in **Table 5-1**.

HMW agents induce an IgE-mediated response with release of preformed and newly formed mediators and subsequent triggering of the characteristic allergic inflammatory response. LMW chemicals may also induce a specific IgE response by forming haptens with body proteins. Other LMW agents may induce a delayed response that may involve a cell-mediated immunologic mechanism [7]. The pathology seen in OA is similar to that seen in nonoccupational asthma, with bronchial wall thickening due to eosinophilic infiltration, edema, smooth muscle hypertrophy, fibroblast proliferation in the subepithelium, and airway obstruction with excessive secretions [2].

Most irritant-induced asthma is caused by LMW chemicals through toxic rather than immunologic mechanisms. In high-level exposures, these agents are thought to cause significant epithelial damage with subsequent onset of neurogenic inflammation via nonadrenergic and noncholinergic pathways. Inflammation may also be triggered by nonspecific activation of macrophages and degranulation of mast cells. Bronchial biopsies have shown epithelial desquamation with lymphocytic exudates that improve after treatment with inhaled corticosteroids. Most patients show histologic recovery, and it is unclear why particular patients continue to have bronchial hyperreactivity [6].

Initial information on the known hazards of some of these agents can be obtained by review of **material safety data sheets (MSDSs)**. The law requires any employer whose company produces or uses hazardous chemicals to keep these sheets on file and to produce them at the request of an employee or health care provider. They contain information on the physical and health hazards of a compound, but they can be cumbersome and even inaccurate [2]. Other resources include the Hazardous Substances Data Bank online database [8], MEDLINE [9], American Conference of Governmental Industrial Hygienists Threshold Limit Values (ACGIH TLV) documentations [10], and the Agency for Toxic Substances and Disease Registry (ATSDR) [11].

Differential Diagnosis

The differential diagnosis includes allergic bronchopulmonary aspergillosis, aspirin idiosyncrasy syndrome, Churg-Strauss vasculitis, vocal cord dysfunction, gastroesophageal reflux disease, congestive heart failure, and hypersensitivity pneumonitis [2,4].

PRESENTATION

Risk Factors

Risk factors for OA include a high degree of exposure to workplace sensitizers, cigarette smoking, and atopy (as demonstrated by positive skin prick tests to common aeroallergens) [5].

History and Physical Exam

The diagnosis of OA requires the physician to produce objective evidence of airflow limitation and/or bronchial hyperresponsiveness and then attempt to causally link this evidence with an exposure found only in the workplace. This begins with a thorough history.

Patients present with complaints of wheezing, dyspnea, chest tightness, or sometimes only a cough. Rhinorrhea, sneezing, sinus congestion, or itching and watering of the eyes may have preceded these symptoms.

**TABLE 5-1. SOME CAUSATIVE AGENTS OF OCCUPATIONAL ASTHMA
GROUPED BY PATHOGENIC MECHANISM**

Mechanism	Type of agent	Causative agent	Occupations
Immunologic IgE-dependent	HMW agents	Animal urine, dander, serum	Lab workers, veterinarians
		Cereal and soy flour	Bakers, millers
		Grain dust	Grain-store workers, farmers
		Enzymes	
		Alpha-amylase, cellulase	Bakers, pharmaceutical workers
		Papain, pepsin	Pharmaceutical and food workers
		Bacillus subtilis– derived, *Aspergillus-* derived	Detergent industry workers
		Gums (acacia, guar)	Printers, carpet manufacturers, hairdressers
		Psyllium	Pharmaceutical workers, nurses
		Egg proteins	Egg-processing workers
		Seeds (cottonseed, linseed, flaxseed)	Bakers, oil producers
		Storage mites	Farmers, grain-store workers
		Latex	Health care workers, manufacturers
Immunologic IgE-dependent	LMW chemicals (haptens)	Acid anhydrides (phthalic, trimellitic)	Plastic, epoxy resin workers
		Platinum salts	Platinum-refinery workers
		Reactive dyes	Textile and dyeing workers
		Persulfate salts	Hairdressers
Immunologic (cell-mediated?)	LMW chemicals	Diisocyanates (toluene, methylene diphenyl, hexamethylene)	Polyurethane, foundry workers, painters
		Western Red Cedar (plicatic acid)	Sawmill workers, carpenters
		Amines	Photographers, shellac workers, chemists
		Colophony	Electronic workers, welders
Nonimmunologic (toxic effect)	LMW chemicals (irritants)	Chlorine	Pulp mill and chemical workers
		Sulfur dioxide	Pyrite workers, miners
		Ammonia	Spray painters, chemical workers
		Sodium fumes	Cleaners, chemical workers
		Smoke	Fire fighters, police officers
		Diisocyanates	Spray painters, polyurethane workers

From Quirce S, Sastre J. Occupational asthma. *Allergy* 1998;53:633–641, with permission from Blackwell/Munksgaard.

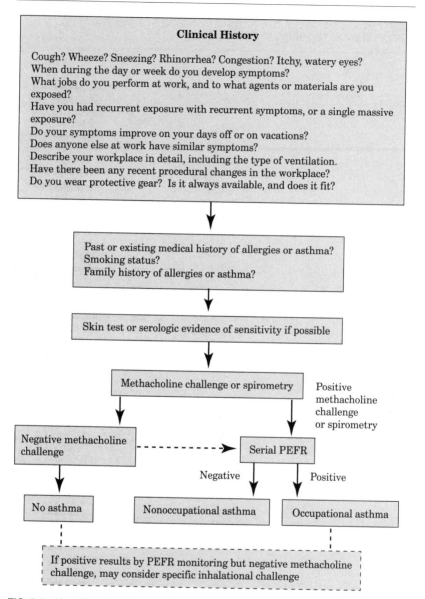

FIG. 5-1. Algorithm for diagnosis of occupational asthma. Mean PEFR consistently reduced by ≥20% with return to baseline when away from work indicates occupational asthma [5].

A detailed job history includes questions (Fig. 5-1) regarding exposures at work, unusual events or spills, whether others at work have similar symptoms, timing of symptoms, and whether there is any improvement away from work. The physician should ask about climatic conditions in the workplace and the use of protective gear.

A medical history should inquire about preexisting asthma, sinusitis, gastroesophageal reflux disease, or other disorders that may confound the diagnosis. Family history of atopic disorders or OA may be helpful, as particular HLA genotypes have been associated with occupational allergy and asthma [12].

Physical exam, lab tests, and imaging studies should be used mainly to exclude other diagnoses considered in the differential diagnosis of OA (see Differential Diagnosis).

Skin prick testing or measurement of specific IgE in the serum may help assess sensitization to a particular agent, but this is available only for a small number of agents involved in OA. Any results must be interpreted in the context of the rest of the clinical evaluation.

MANAGEMENT

Diagnosis

Diagnostic evaluation continues with the objective diagnosis of asthma.

Reversible airflow limitation may be demonstrated by spirometry, or nonspecific bronchial hyperreactivity may be established by methacholine or histamine challenge. A positive test only establishes bronchial reactivity, not its etiology.

The clinician must then establish a temporal relationship between workplace exposure and symptoms. The standard method is by **serial measurement of peak expiratory flow rates (PEFRs)**. Although this method is limited by problems with compliance and precision, it has been found to be 96% sensitive and 89% specific for OA in one study [2]. Four measurements (morning, midshift, after work, and at bedtime) are recommended over a 2-wk period. Ideally, this should be compared to a 1- to 2-wk period away from work [2]. Issues of compliance and accuracy can now be addressed with self-recording peak flow meters and computerized hand-held spirometers.

A specific inhalational challenge remains the gold standard for diagnosis of IgE-mediated OA, as it is the closest one can come to establishing a causal link between a workplace exposure and the patient's symptoms. This procedure may be most useful in cases of discordance between clinical history or PEFR monitoring and measurement of bronchial hyperreactivity. The challenge may be performed in the lab or in the workplace but requires the presence of trained personnel and emergency equipment. Its use has mainly been limited to large regional surveillance programs [2].

The diagnosis of RADS is less clear cut. Major and minor criteria for diagnosis have been used and are given in reference 6.

Treatment

OA treatment primarily involves **avoidance of triggers**. Proper diagnosis of OA is vital, as it may require removal of a worker from the workplace. Pharmaceutical treatment with bronchodilators and inhaled corticosteroids may also be required.

KEY POINTS

- OA is defined as variable airflow limitation and/or bronchial hyperresponsiveness caused by workplace exposures.
- The treatment of OA requires avoidance of workplace triggers.

REFERENCES

1. Bernstein IL, Chan-Yeung M, Malo J-L, Bernstein D, eds. *Asthma in the workplace*. New York: Marcel Dekker, 1993.
2. Rabatin J, Cowl C. A guide to the diagnosis and treatment of occupational asthma. *Mayo Clin Proc* 2001;76:633–640.
3. Meredith S. Occupational asthma: measures of frequency from four countries. *Thorax* 1996;51:435–440.

4. Mihilas L. An approach to the diagnosis of occupational asthma. *Ann Allergy Asthma Immunol* 1999;83:577–582.
5. Bernstein D. Allergic reactions to workplace allergens. *JAMA* 1997;278:1907–1913.
6. Bardana E. Reactive airways dysfunction syndrome (RADS): guidelines for diagnosis and treatment and insight into likely prognosis. *Ann Allergy Asthma Immunol* 1999;83:583–586.
7. Mapp C, Boschetto P, Miotto D, et al. Mechanisms of occupational asthma. *Ann Allergy Asthma Immunol* 1999;83:645–664.
8. Hazardous Substances Data Bank (TOXNET database online). http://toxnet.nlm.nih.gov. Bethesda, MD: National Library of Medicine.
9. MEDLINE (database online). http://www.ncbi.nlm.nih.gov/entrez/query.fcgi. Bethesda, MD: National Library of Medicine.
10. American Conference of Governmental Industrial Hygienists (ACGIH). *1998 TLVs and BEIs: documentations for threshold limit values for chemical substances and physical agents*. Cincinnati: ACGIH, 1998.
11. Agency for Toxic Substances and Disease Registry. Toxicological profiles. Atlanta: U.S. Department of Health and Human Services.
12. Quirce S, Sastre J. Occupational asthma. *Allergy* 1998;53:633–641.

Hypersensitivity Pneumonitis

Alpa L. Jani

INTRODUCTION

Hypersensitivity pneumonitis (HP), also termed *extrinsic allergic alveolitis*, is an immunologically mediated alveolitis caused by exposure to various antigens in a susceptible host. It is a clinical diagnosis based on a combination of historical, radiographic, and lab findings. Its presentation in the acute or subacute form may be confused with atypical pneumonia or with other types of interstitial lung disease, such as sarcoidosis. In the chronic form, it may appear similar to other causes of pulmonary fibrosis.

Epidemiology

The greatest **risk factor** for HP is exposure to a causative antigen (Table 6-1). As prevalence of disease varies in exposed populations, host susceptibility factors must also play a role, but these factors have not been well delineated. Neither atopy nor specific HLA genotypes have any clear association with disease. HP does occur with lesser frequency in cigarette smokers as compared to nonsmokers [1].

The **prevalence** of HP varies by antigen. The most common types in the United States include farmer's lung, caused by thermophilic actinomyces; bird breeder's lung, caused by avian proteins; ventilation pneumonitis, caused by molds or amoeba; and chemical worker's lung, caused by low-molecular-weight (LMW) chemicals [2,3]. Estimates of the prevalence of farmer's lung range from 2–8%, with newer reports citing a lower prevalence likely due to changes in farming practices. The prevalence of pigeon breeder's lung is reported as 6–21% of those exposed. In HP from antigens found in ventilation and humidification systems, the prevalence has been reported to be as high as 15% among those exposed [4].

CAUSES

Pathophysiology

Etiologic Agents

Etiologic agents that cause HP are many and varied (Table 6-1). These agents can be divided into organic high-molecular-weight antigens and LMW chemicals [4]. Among the organic antigens are the thermophilic actinomycetes that grow in "moldy" hay or sugar cane, animal proteins such as those found in the excreta or secreta of birds, molds that grow in wood dust, and amoeba found in ventilation systems. LMW chemicals include diisocyanates used in paints and acid anhydrides used in the production of plastics. These chemicals act as antigens by forming haptens with body proteins.

Pathology

The acute form of HP is characterized by alveolar and terminal bronchiolar inflammation consisting initially of neutrophils followed by an increase in lymphocytes, acti-

TABLE 6-1. EXAMPLES OF ETIOLOGIC AGENTS IN HYPERSENSITIVITY PNEUMONITIS

Antigen	Exposure	Disease
High-molecular-weight antigens		
Thermophilic actinomycetes		
Thermoactinomyces vulgaris, T. viridis	Moldy hay	Farmer's lung
T. sacchari, T. vulgaris	Moldy sugar cane	Bagassosis
Molds		
Aspergillus clavatus	Moldy barley	Malt worker's disease
Alternaria	Oak, cedar, and mahogany dust; pine and spruce pulp	Woodworker's lung
Penicillium	Moldy cork dust	Suberosis
Pullularia	Moldy sequoia dust	Sequoiosis
Animal		
Glycoprotein [4]	Droppings or feathers of pigeon, parakeet, chicken, turkey, goose, owl, dove, duck	Bird fancier's, breeder's, or handler's lung
Antigen in rat urine	Lab rat	Lab worker's hypersensitivity pneumonitis
Acanthamoeba castellani, Naegleria gruberi [4]	Contaminated water in humidification and forced-air conditioning systems	Ventilation pneumonitis, or humidifier lung
Low-molecular-weight chemicals		
Hexamethylene diisocyanate	Refinishing agents	Bathtub finisher's lung
Trimellitic anhydride, phthalic anhydride	Plastics	Plastic worker's lung, late respiratory systemic syndrome [4]

vated macrophages, and plasma cells. CD8$^+$ T lymphocytes outnumber CD4$^+$ T lymphocytes in this inflammatory cell infiltrate [4].

In the subacute form, noncaseating granulomata are seen. These are less well organized than those found in sarcoidosis. These granulomata may persist or disappear in the chronic form of HP, which shows interstitial fibrosis, mainly in the upper zones of the lung [1].

Immunology

Although precipitating antibody in the serum is characteristically associated with HP, a specific mechanism of hypersensitivity has been difficult to assign [4].

A type III, or immune complex–mediated, form of hypersensitivity was initially regarded as the major mechanism of hypersensitivity in HP. Supporting this theory is the development of symptoms several hours to days after exposure, and the finding of increased levels of Ig and complement in bronchoalveolar lavage (BAL) fluid and lung lesions [1].

Newer evidence from animal models of HP points to the role of a **type IV** (delayed-type) **hypersensitivity** mechanism. In these animal models, HP has been passively transferred using sensitized lymphocytes followed by respiratory tract challenge. However, with hyperimmune serum, it has been difficult to generate this disease, arguing against the role of circulating antibodies. Also, agents that inhibit cell-mediated hypersensitivity inhibit granuloma formation in these models [1].

Regardless of the initial mechanism of hypersensitivity, the central event in HP is thought to be an exposure to a causative antigen followed by **granulomatous inflammation**. This inflammation is then modulated by cytokines and suppressor factors [1]. Support for the latter comes from patients with pigeon breeder's lung, who appear to have a defect in the suppressor function of the CD8$^+$ cells found in BAL fluid [4].

Differential Diagnosis

Differentiation of HP from other interstitial lung diseases requires taking a thorough **exposure history** and using the tests mentioned above to gather the necessary objective information.

The exposure history should include a listing of occupations and hobbies, both present and past. Exposure to farm or domestic animals and fowl should be documented.

All **medications** the patient is taking should be examined to rule out a drug-induced lung disease.

Any evidence of **systemic disease** that may raise suspicion for a collagen vascular disorder should be thoroughly investigated.

Eosinophilic pneumonia and allergic bronchopulmonary aspergillosis should be distinguished from HP by their association with asthma (with an obstructive rather than restrictive pattern on pulmonary function testing), and eosinophilia, which is not a feature of HP.

Sarcoidosis may be distinguished from HP by a predominance of CD4$^+$ lymphocytes in BAL fluid, and possibly by hilar lymph node or multi-organ involvement. BAL fluid may also help to distinguish the chronic form of HP from idiopathic pulmonary fibrosis, which is associated with a predominance of neutrophils in the lavage fluid [3].

The acute form of HP is sometimes confused with the organic dust toxic syndrome (ODTS), a distinct entity that is significantly more common than farmer's lung [5]. ODTS presents with transient fever and muscle aches acutely after heavy exposure to organic dust. Unlike in farmer's lung, serum precipitins can be absent, and chest x-ray and spirometry are normal. ODTS has no immunologic basis and is a self-limited disorder [3].

PRESENTATION

Clinical Presentation

HP generally presents as an **interstitial pneumonitis** in an acute, subacute, or chronic form.

The acute form of HP manifests with cough, fever, chills, and dyspnea occurring 6–8 hrs after exposure, with resolution of symptoms in 1–2 days, as long as antigen exposure ceases.

The subacute form of disease presents several weeks after exposure with cough and progressive dyspnea. Again, as long as antigen exposure ceases, the manifestations of HP in the subacute form should disappear.

If antigen exposure continues, however, the chronic form of HP may ensue. A patient may experience continued cough, dyspnea, and weight loss. With chronic low-level exposure, the chronic form of HP may present with new-onset exertional dyspnea without a past history of acute or subacute disease [3].

MANAGEMENT

Diagnosis

Neutrophilia and lymphopenia may be present after acute exposure [3]. Neither eosinophilia nor elevation of IgE is a specific feature of HP.

A **chest x-ray** may be normal or may show discrete nodular or diffuse poorly defined infiltrates in the acute or subacute form of the disease. In the chronic form, reticulonodular infiltrates, fibrosis, or honeycombing are seen. Thus, there is no particular chest x-ray finding that is unique to HP. High-resolution chest CT scan may show diffuse lung involvement with prominence of medium-sized bronchial walls and patchy areas of reticular and nodular alveolar infiltrate in the midzone of the lung, with absence of hilar lymph node enlargement [3]. However, these findings are not pathognomonic for HP.

Almost all symptomatic patients with HP have **precipitating antibody** to the antigen of exposure [4]. These antibodies are usually detected by immunoprecipitation (Ouchterlony gel immunodiffusion). However, the diagnosis of HP cannot rest on the presence of these serum precipitins, as asymptomatic individuals may also have a positive test for such precipitins without ever exhibiting symptoms of HP. Conversely, false-negative serum precipitins may result from poor-quality antigens [3] or from sera with high antibody titer [4].

Pulmonary function testing typically reveals a restrictive pattern, impaired diffusion capacity, and exercise-induced hypoxemia. An obstructive pattern may develop in the chronic stage and lead to a mixed pattern on pulmonary function testing.

BAL may be helpful in diagnosis, showing increased lymphocytes with a predominance of $CD8^+$ cells relative to $CD4^+$ cells. Lung biopsy is usually not required for diagnosis but sometimes may be performed in the acute form when the etiology cannot be distinguished from other causes of fever with cough and pulmonary infiltrates [3].

Skin testing and provocational challenge are reserved mostly for the research setting.

Treatment

Treatment of all forms of HP requires **avoidance** of antigen exposure.

For some exposures, avoidance of antigen exposure may be as simple as the removal of a house pet, but in other cases, avoidance requires a drastic change in the life and livelihood of the patient. Thus, complete antigen avoidance may be difficult to achieve, and environmental control may become a focus of treatment. This may include advising the patient not to bale or store hay when it is wet or to wear a pollen mask, personal respirator, or ventilated helmet with any exposure to antigen. A mask must efficiently remove particles of 0.2–10 μm in size to be effective [2]. In the case of ventilation pneumonitis, replacement of the contaminated portion of the ventilation system may be necessary.

Treatment with **prednisone (Deltasone)** at 1 mg/kg/day or its equivalent for 7–14 days may be indicated in the subacute form of HP. This dose may be tapered over 2–6 wks as tolerated. Even patients with the chronic form of HP may benefit from a trial of corticosteroids at similar doses for 2–4 wks to obtain maximal reversibility of their disease. Corticosteroids should then be tapered to the lowest dose tolerated [3].

Specific predictors of progression to chronic disease have not been identified. Curiously, some patients may progress to chronic disease without continued antigen exposure, and yet others may have resolution of disease despite continued antigen exposure [6].

Long-term mortality for patients with the chronic form of HP is estimated to be 3–9% [2]. Corticosteroid treatment does not appear to have an effect on this long-term outcome [3,6].

KEY POINTS

- HP is an immunologically mediated alveolitis caused by exposure to various organic antigens and LMW chemicals.

- HP should be considered in the differential diagnosis of fever, cough, and pulmonary infiltrates.
- Treatment of HP requires avoidance of antigen exposure and may involve the use of corticosteroids.

REFERENCES

1. Salvaggio JE. Extrinsic allergic alveolitis (hypersensitivity pneumonitis): past, present, and future. *Clin Exp Allergy* 1997;27(Supp 1):18–25.
2. Pitcher WD. Southwestern Internal Medicine Conference: hypersensitivity pneumonitis. *Am J Med Sci* 1990;300:251–266.
3. Kline JN, Hunninghake GW. Hypersensitivity pneumonitis and pulmonary infiltrates with eosinophilia. In: Braunwald E, Fauci A, Kasper D, et al., eds. *Harrison's principles of internal medicine*, 15th ed. New York: McGraw-Hill, 2001; 1463–1467.
4. Grammer LC. Occupational allergic alveolitis. *Ann Allergy Asthma Immunol* 1999;83:602–606.
5. Von Essen S, Fryzek J, Nowakowski B, et al. Respiratory symptoms and farming practices in farmers associated with an acute febrile illness after organic dust exposure. *Chest* 1999;116:1452–1458.
6. Rose C, King TE. Controversies in hypersensitivity pneumonitis. *Am Rev Respir Dis* 1992;145:1–2.

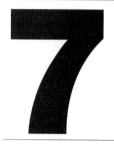

Pulmonary Function Tests

Shirley S. Joo

INTRODUCTION

Pulmonary function tests (PFTs) are valuable adjuncts to treatment and assessment of respiratory diseases. Common tools used in clinical practice include PFTs, bronchoprovocation testing, and the peak flow meter.

PULMONARY FUNCTION TESTS

PFTs help to assess the static and dynamic components of a patient's lung function and usually include four types of measurements: spirometry, lung volumes, lung diffusion capacity, and flow volume loops. An algorithm for interpretation of PFTs is given in Fig. 7-1.

Spirometry

Spirometry is very much a **patient effort–dependent test** that requires the understanding and cooperation of patients for accurate and reproducible test results. The test can be performed with either closed-circuit spirometry or an open-circuit system. Both are equally reliable and have some different advantages and disadvantages. The closed circuit allows more accurate measurement of the functional residual capacity (FRC), but because the patient breathes into the machine, maintaining good hygiene is a concern. To obtain acceptable test results, guidelines published by the American Thoracic Society should be followed. The minimum number of respiratory loops needed is three, and the best forced expiratory volume in 1 sec (FEV_1) and forced vital capacity (FVC) of the three test values should be recorded and used for interpretation. The maximum recommended number for consecutive testing is eight, because studies have shown that patient fatigue becomes a significant factor after more than eight trials [1].

Traditional spirometry measures lung volumes using a water-sealed chamber. It is expressed as change in lung volume over time. A more modern method using an electronic device measures flow rate as a function of lung volume during inspiration and expiration. The flow volume loop can be invaluable in difficult diagnostic cases by providing insight into functional characteristics of upper and lower airways as well as possible functional defects due to extrathoracic causes.

Indications
DIAGNOSTIC

- Evaluate presence of pulmonary disease
- Evaluate symptoms of dyspnea, cough, or wheezing
- Screen for high-risk individuals (e.g., smokers or those with occupational exposures)
- Preop evaluation

MONITORING

- Assess response to bronchodilator therapy

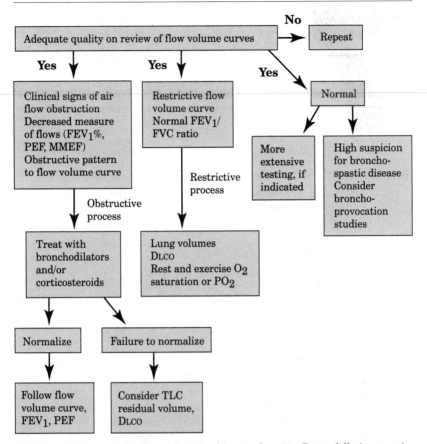

FIG. 7-1. Algorithm for interpretation of pulmonary function. DLCO, diffusion capacity of lung for carbon monoxide; FEV_1, forced expiratory volume in 1 sec; FVC, forced vital capacity; MMEF, maximal mid expiratory flow; PEF, peak expiratory flow; PO_2, partial pressure of oxygen; TLC, total lung capacity.

- Follow progression of present pulmonary disease
- Assess for adverse reactions to drugs that may have pulmonary side effects (e.g., amiodarone)
- Assess pulmonary dysfunction in response to environmental exposures

    OTHER

- Documentation of disability for insurance
- Assess for qualifications for rehabilitation programs

Criteria for Acceptable Spirometry

Criteria for acceptable spirometry from the American Thoracic Society are (a) a smooth continuous exhalation for >6 secs demonstrating a *plateau*, defined as no change in the volume for at least 1 sec during expiration; (b) a satisfactory start of test without hesitation or false start; (c) lack of artifacts such as coughing, glottic closure, early termination of exhalation, or obstructed mouth piece; and (d) properly calibrated equipment without leak [2].

Criteria for Reproducibility

The reproducibility of lung function tests are important not only for following the longitudinal trends but also to ensure that such tests can be compared from one test center to the another. These criteria are that (a) the largest FVC should be within 0.2 L of the second largest FVC value, and (b) the largest FEV_1 should be within 0.2 L of the second largest FEV_1. Additional spirograms (maximum of eight) should be obtained to assure that the above criteria are met in at least three of the maneuvers [2].

Frequency

Follow-up spirograms are used mainly for monitoring purposes and can be repeated at the physician's discretion. For asthma patients, guidelines recommend an initial diagnostic spirogram and at least one annually for management of therapy.

Values Derived from Spirometry

- FVC: the volume of gas that can be forcefully expelled after maximal inhalation
- FEV_1: the volume measured in the first sec of maximal forced exhalation
- $FEF_{25-75\%}$: maximal mid expiratory flow rate; flow during 25–75% of vital capacity
- PEF (peak expiratory flow) or FEF max: maximal airflow rate achieved during expiration

Measured Lung Volumes

- TLC (total lung capacity): volume of lungs after maximal inspiration
- VC (vital capacity): volume of gas measured with slow expiration after maximal inhalation
- FRC: volume left in lungs after normal exhalation (TLC – inspiratory capacity)

Other Values and Tests

- ABG: arterial blood gas
- DLCO: diffusion capacity between capillary and alveolar wall using CO

Airway Obstruction

Airway obstruction is an important diagnosis made using PFTs. When airway obstruction is present, the values of FEV_1 and FVC are both reduced, but FEV_1 is disproportionately reduced compared to FVC, thus giving a lower FEV_1:FVC ratio. The primary criterion for diagnosis of obstruction is FEV_1:FVC <87% of predicted. Occasionally, in the face of borderline FEV_1/FVC, earlier airflow obstruction may be detected by $FEF_{25-75\%}$, the rationale being that earlier changes in airway obstruction start in the smaller and peripheral airways. However, this is a nonspecific finding and should not be used as a criterion for diagnosis of small airways disease. The severity of airway obstruction is graded on predicted FEV.

ASTHMA. The primary functional abnormality is the presence of reversible airway obstruction. This can be demonstrated on spirometry by measurement of FEV_1 and FVC before and after administration of bronchodilators. Reversibilty of >12% of FEV_1 (or 200 cc increase from baseline) is diagnostic for asthma. However, the absence of improvement after bronchodilator treatment does not exclude reversible obstruction. The obstruction may be due to inflammation, which may only be reversible after prolonged antiinflammatory therapy. Another confounding problem is that some COPD patients will have reversible airway obstruction as a component of their disease. The DLCO, which is normal in asthma but increased or decreased in other obstructive diseases, can somtimes help to differentiate COPD from asthma. (*See Table 7-1 for sample PFTs of a patient with asthma.*)

EMPHYSEMA/COPD. The functional defect in emphysema is an obstructive picture with reduction in the ratio of FEV_1: FVC, which is usually not responsive to bronchodilator therapy. The DLCO is reduced, and static lung compliance is increased. Later in the disease, as air trapping becomes more evident, the TLC and residual volume (RV) increase, resulting in an increase in the RV:TLC ratio. (*See Table 7-2 for sample PFTs of a patient with emphysema/COPD.*)

TABLE 7-1. SAMPLE PULMONARY FUNCTION TESTS (PFTs) OF A PATIENT WITH ASTHMA

| PFT | Before bronchodilator | | After bronchodilator | | |
	Actual	% Predicted	Actual	% Predicted	% Change
FVC (L)	3.14	67	4.32	92	25
FEV_1 (L)	2.12	53	3.24	81	28
FEV_1/FVC (%)		67		75	
$FEF_{25-75\%}$ (L/sec)	0.63	14	1.43	33	
TLC (L)	6.45	100			
DLCO (mL/min/ mm Hg)	32	100			

DLCO, diffusion capacity of lung for carbon monoxide; $FEF_{25-75\%}$, maximal mid expiratory rate; FEV_1, forced expiratory volume in 1 sec; FVC, forced vital capacity; TLC, total lung capacity.

Restrictive Lung Disease

The primary defect in restrictive lung disease is a decreased TLC <70% of predicted. The FEV_1 and FVC are usually proportionately reduced and, therefore, will give a normal ratio of FEV_1:FVC. As the disease process progresses, FVC may decrease faster than FEV_1 and, thus, can increase the ratio. (*See Table 7-3 for sample PFTs of a patient with restrictive lung disease.*) Severity of restrictive defect is graded based on the amount of decrease of TLC or VC.

BRONCHOPROVOCATION TESTING

Bronchial hyperresponsiveness (BHR) is a hallmark feature of asthma that is demonstrable in nearly all patients with asthma. BHR can be measured via bronchoprovocation with agents known to cause bronchial constriction.

TABLE 7-2. SAMPLE PULMONARY FUNCTION TESTS (PFTS) OF A PATIENT WITH EMPHYSEMA/CHRONIC OBSTRUCTIVE PULMONARY DISEASE

| PFT | Before bronchodilator | | After bronchodilator | | |
	Actual	% Predicted	Actual	% Predicted	% Change
FVC (L)	2.5	62	2.5	62	0
FEV_1 (L)	1.58	50	1.44	46	-4
FEV_1/FVC (%)		63		57	
$FEF_{25-75\%}$ (L/sec)	1.3	33	1.3	0	
RV (L)	4	160			
TLC (L)	7.12	110			
DLCO (mL/min/mm Hg)	25	78			

DLCO, diffusion capacity of lung for carbon monoxide; $FEF_{25-75\%}$, maximal mid expiratory rate; FEV_1, forced expiratory volume in 1 sec; FVC, forced vital capacity; RV, residual volume; TLC, total lung capacity.

TABLE 7-3. SAMPLE PULMONARY FUNCTION TESTS (PFTS) OF A PATIENT WITH RESTRICTIVE LUNG DISEASE

PFT	Actual	% Predicted
FVC (L)	1.8	45
FEV_1 (L)	1.62	47
FEV_1/FVC (%)	90	
$FEF_{25-75\%}$ (L/sec)	1.4	41
TLC (L)	4.16	65

$FEF_{25-75\%}$, maximal mid expiratory rate; FEV_1, forced expiratory volume in 1 sec; FVC, forced vital capacity; TLC, total lung capacity.

Methacholine and histamine challenges are the two most widely used methods of testing BHR. Both agents are equally effective, but methacholine is the agent of choice among many clinicians, because histamine has more systemic side effects, such as headache, tachycardia, and flushing. Another disadvantage to histamine is that tachyphylaxis can develop at higher concentrations and with consecutive repeated exposures. Provocholine is an FDA-approved, commercially available methacholine widely used in clinical settings because it is easier to store and meets quality and consistency standards.

Indications

- Suspicion of asthma by history but nondiagnostic PFTs
- Assessing the relative risk for developing occupational asthma
- Evaluation of severity of occupational asthma

Contraindications

Absolute Contraindications

- Severe airflow obstruction (FEV_1 <50% predicted or <1 L)
- Myocardial infarction or CVA within 3 mos
- Uncontrolled HTN with systolic BP >200 or diastolic BP >100
- Known aortic aneurysm

Relative Contraindications

- Moderate airflow obstruction (FEV_1 <60% predicted or <1.5 L)
- Inability to cooperate or follow directions for test
- Pregnancy
- Breast feeding
- Current use of cholinesterase inhibitor medication

These relative contraindications are because methacholine is a class C drug in pregnancy. See Table 7-4 for a list of drugs to withhold before bronchoprovocation testing.

Methods

There are two widely used protocols for bronchoprovocation.

Two-Minute Tidal Breathing Protocol

For the 2-min tidal breathing protocol, the patient is given each dose via nebulizer and should breathe tidal breaths for exactly 2 mins. FEV_1 is measured at end of each 2

**TABLE 7-4. MEDICATIONS TO WITHHOLD BEFORE
BRONCHOPROVOCATION TESTING**

Medication name	Minimum interval from last dose
Short-acting beta agonist	
Albuterol	8 hrs
Ipratropium	24 hrs
Long-acting inhaled bronchodilator	
Salmeterol, formoterol	48 hrs
Oral bronchodilators	
Theophyllines	12 hrs
Intermediate theophylline	24 hrs
Long-acting theophylline	48 hrs
Standard beta agonist tablet	12 hrs
Long-acting beta agonist tablet	24 hrs
Cromolyn sodium	8 hrs
Nedocromil	48 hrs
Hydroxyzine, cetirizine	3 days
Leukotriene modifiers	24 hrs
Caffeine	Day of study

Reprinted from Crapo RO, Casaburi R, Coates AL, et al. Guidelines for methacholine and exercise challenge testing, 1999. *Am J Respir Crit Care Med* 2000;161:309–329, with permission from American Thoracic Society.

mins, and the highest FEV_1 from the acceptable volume loops is recorded. If the FEV_1 changes by <20% from the baseline, then the next dose is given. However, if the FEV_1 changes by >20% from baseline, then the test is terminated, and patient should be assessed for symptoms. At the conclusion of the test, inhaled albuterol is administered, and after 10 mins, repeat spirometry is obtained.

Five-Breath Dosimeter Protocol
For this method, the subject is given a nebulizer with dosimeter attached. The first concentration is placed in the nebulizer, and after complete exhalation, the patient takes a slow (5-sec), deep breath through the mouthpiece. As soon as the first slow breath is initiated, the dosimeter is started to administer the methacholine. The patient continues to take slow, deep breaths consecutively for a total of 5 breaths, which should be completed in 2 mins. FEV_1 is measured approximately 30 secs and 90 secs after the fifth inhalation. These maneuvers are repeated until FEV_1 decreases by >20% or the maximal concentration is reached. Once the test is terminated, inhaled albuterol is administered, and spirometry is repeated 10 mins later.

Measurement of Response
Measurement of response to the bronchial challenge can be expressed in various ways. These include reporting the decrease in FEV_1, airways resistance, maximum expiratory flow volume curves, or total respiratory resistance. The most used method in clinical practice is the measurement of decrease in FEV_1. This is reported in conjunction with PC_{20}, which is defined as the concentration of constrictor agent at which FEV_1 falls by 20% from baseline. A decrease in FEV_1 by

20% is, by definition, considered a statistically significant change signifying airway hyperresponsiveness.

Positive Test Result

Positive test results are usually defined as a PC_{20} <8 mg/mL or 16 mg/mL, because methacholine is a nonspecific bronchoconstrictor and can lead to bronchoconstriction in all people when given in high enough doses. Whether the patient should be diagnosed with asthma requires critical assessment of the pretest probability and clinical suspicion. Asthmatic patients usually have a positive response at concentrations lower than 8 mg/mL.

Negative Test Result

A *negative test result* is defined as absence of bronchial constriction at concentration >16 mg/mL. A negative test has a higher predictive value and rules out the diagnosis of asthma.

Bronchial Inhalation Challenge with Antigen

When an extrinsic allergen is suspected as a source for bronchial hyperresponsiveness based on skin testing or radioallergosorbent assay test, inhalation challenge with the allergens can be used to confirm the suspicion. Bronchial challenge can help to clarify the role of the extrinsic allergen in asthma and to convince patients of the cause-effect relationship of their disease. Otherwise, it is done primarily for research purposes when evaluating new treatment modalities and mediator-blocking agents.

PEAK FLOW METERS

Peak expiratory flow rates (PEFRs) can be calculated from a spirogram or measured with a hand-held peak flow meter. Peak expiratory flows can be used roughly to diagnose asthma; however, this is not recommended practice. The PEFR is useful as an outpatient tool in measuring response to therapy as well as monitoring for early symptoms of exacerbation or helping to identify provocative factors.

Normal values of PEFR are based on age, gender, and height. In addition, there is a well-documented diurnal variation to the peak flow values, with lowest values occurring in the early morning on awakening and highest values obtained during 4–6 P.M. It is important to obtain values in the mornings and the evenings. Each measurement should be the highest value from three consecutive maneuvers. If there is 20% diurnal variation, this is a suggestion of airway hyperresponsiveness, and further treatment or testing should be instituted.

Studies have shown that adult patients are able to correctly identify symptom exacerbations before a decrease in the peak flow meter values; however, pediatric patients and their parents report being symptom free until the peak expiratory flow values are in the worrisome range. Peak flow meters provide some valuable objective measurements to follow and tailor therapy. Alert values are usually divided into three zones: green, yellow, and red (see Chap. 3, Allergic Rhinitis and Sinusitis). The yellow zone indicates mild symptoms and is marked at 80% below the patient's predicted maximal PEFR. This usually signals need for contacting a physician and possible escalation of treatment, either with an increasing dose of beta agonist, a course of antibiotics, adjustment of other medications, or a course of oral corticosteroids.

VOCAL CORD DYSFUNCTION

Vocal cord dysfunction (VCD) is a disease that can mimic the diagnosis of asthma and can coexist with asthma. VCD should be considered especially in patients with diagnosis of asthma but who have no clinical improvement in response to escalating bronchodilator or corticosteroid therapy. Epidemiologic studies show that VCD is most prevalent among female patients between the ages of 20–40.

Symptoms

Symptoms of VCD include wheezing, dyspnea, throat tightness, and voice change.

Diagnosis

Diagnosis can be made either by PFTs or by fiberoptic rhinolaryngoscopy. PFTs may show abnormalities of blunting or truncation of the inspiratory portion of the flow volume loop. The best method of diagnosis, however, is by direct visualization of the vocal cords using fiberoptic rhinolaryngoscopy during inspiration and expiration. The pathognomonic finding in VCD is anterior adduction of the vocal cords while the posterior portion of the vocal cords remains open during inspiration.

Treatment

Treatment for VCD has been breathing exercise and voice training to decrease laryngeal muscle tone. These techniques can be taught by a trained speech therapist. Medications to treat asthma, such as bronchodilators and corticosteroids, may be useful in patients with VCD and asthma, but there is a definite tendency for these patients to overuse asthma medications. In pure VCD patients, asthma medications are not useful and may even be deleterious.

KEY POINTS

- PFTs are a good diagnostic tool and are also helpful in assessing the severity of lung disease and in guiding therapy.
- In obstructive lung disease, FEV_1 is disproportionately reduced compared to FVC, thus giving a lower FEV_1/FVC ratio.
- The primary defect in restrictive lung disease is a decrease in TLC $<70\%$ of predicted.
- Reversibility of FEV_1 by $>12\%$ is diagnostic of asthma.
- VCD should be considered in patients with diagnosis of asthma but no clinical improvement despite escalating medical therapy.

SUGGESTED READING

Crapo RO, Casaburi R, Coates AL, et al. Guidelines for Methacholine and Exercise Challenge Testing-1999. This official statement of the American Thoracic Society was adopted by the ATS Board of Directors, July 1999. *Am J Respir Crit Care Med* 2000;161:309–329.

Cross D, Nelson HS. The role of the peak flow meter in the diagnosis and management of asthma. *J Allergy Clin Immunol* 1991;87:176–184.

Nelson HS. Asthma guidelines and outcomes. In: Middleton E, ed. *Allergy: principles and practice*, 5th ed. St. Louis: Mosby, 1998;927–937.

Wood RP, Milgrom H. Vocal cord dysfunction [review article]. *J Allergy Clin Immunol* 1996;98(3):481–485.

REFERENCES

1. American Thoracic Society. Lung function testing: selection of references values and interpretive strategies. *Am Rev Respir Dis* 1991;144:1202–1218.
2. American Thoracic Society. Standardization of spirometry. *Am J Respir Crit Care Med* 1995;152:1107–1136.

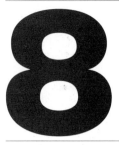

In Vivo and *In Vitro* Diagnostic Tests for Allergy

Shirley S. Joo

INTRODUCTION

Since the characterization of IgE and its role in the pathophysiology of allergic symptoms, many clinical tests have been used to help detect specific antigen sensitivities. Two types of tests are widely used to detect the presence of IgE. One is skin testing, and the other is the *in vitro* measurement of IgE. Both tests, however, are only adjuncts to thorough exposure history that indicates the presence of relevant IgE-mediated symptoms or signs and the physical exam.

METHODS OF SKIN TESTS

Immediate Hypersensitivity Skin Testing

Immediate hypersensitivity skin testing is the most sensitive and cost-effective method to screen existing IgE sensitivities that may be responsible for clinical symptoms. The antigen is directly applied to the skin surface by different methods. One is epicutaneous, and the other is intradermal. The response recorded is due to immediate hypersensitivity, which is primarily a histamine response and manifests with induration and erythema, the "wheal and flare" reaction. Skin testing should be performed by a trained professional who is familiar with possible adverse reactions and the implications of a positive or a negative test result as it relates to the patient's symptom history and clinical picture.

Indications

- Documentation of allergic sensitivity to specific allergens in patients with asthma, rhinitis, eczema, food allergy, drug allergy, or insect hypersensitivity.
- Monitoring of immunotherapy effects.

Contraindications

- Skin tests should not be performed in patients who have had a recent severe allergic reaction (e.g., anaphylaxis), because test results are unreliable in these instances. Skin testing is usually postponed for 4–6 wks after the acute event.
- Tests should not be performed on patients who have severe eczema or dermatographism because of difficulty in interpreting the results.
- Skin testing should be performed with extreme caution in patients with a history of severe hypersensitivity reactions (e.g., to venom, foods, drugs) and usually not while patients are on beta-adrenergic blocking agents.

Medications to Avoid before Skin Testing

Several medications can interfere with skin testing results. Antihistamines, both H_1 and H_2 blockers, should be discontinued for >72 hrs; fexofenadine (Allegra) for

5–7 days; loratadine (Claritin) for 7 days; and cetirizine (Zyrtec) for 7–10 days. Tricyclic antidepressants (e.g., doxepin), which can have antihistaminic effects, should also be discontinued for 1 wk (taper if necessary!). Some atypical antipsychotic agents (e.g., risperidone, olanzapine, ziprasidone) also have antihistaminic effects and may interfere with skin testing. Beta-blockers, in almost all instances, should be discontinued for ≥24 hrs, because they may increase the risk of a severe allergic reaction.

Epicutaneous Skin Tests

Epicutaneous skin tests include prick and puncture techniques. These methods introduce the antigen into the epidermis of the skin and thereby activate any IgE-sensitized mast cells by the cross-linking of IgE molecules present on the mast cell surface. This, in turn, releases mediators from the mast cell, including histamine, tryptase, chymase, and heparin. Typically, the local reaction will be detectable by wheal and flare reaction within 15 mins. However, some sensitivities are not detectable by this method, and further testing (i.e., intradermal skin tests [see below]) is needed. Preferred areas for testing are the back and volar aspect of the arm.

Prick Skin Test
The prick skin test is performed by placing a small drop of allergen on the cleansed skin surface and passing a 25- or 26-gauge needle through the antigen at a 45-degree angle. The needle should be lightly pressed into the epidermis and then lifted, creating a break in the epidermis without causing bleeding. Test antigens should be placed >2 cm from one another. Various hollow and solid bore needles and blood lancets are available under different trade names.

Puncture Skin Test
The puncture skin test is performed by placing a small drop of the allergen extract on the cleansed skin surface and then puncturing the skin with a device at a perpendicular angle, penetrating 1–1.5 mm into the skin. Commercially available devices made of plastic allow for placement of multiple antigen test sites at one time. Each test antigen site should be placed >2 cm apart. Devices include the Allersharp (previously known as Morrow-Brown Allergy needle) needle (Quorum Allergy, Mississauga, Ontario), Multi-Test II (Lincoln Diagnostics, Inc., Decatur, IL), and DermaPIKII (Biomedex, Spokane, WA). The Multi-Test II requires a slightly different technique, in that the allergen extract is placed on the prongs before it is used to puncture the skin.

Scratch Skin Test
The scratch skin test is performed by making abrasions on the skin and then applying the allergen extract to the site, allowing it to diffuse through the skin. Because of its poor standardization and reproducibility, this method has fallen out of favor and is rarely used.

Intradermal Skin Testing

Intradermal skin testing is more sensitive than the epicutaneous skin tests, but it is generally only performed if the epicutaneous test is negative. The test is performed using 25- to 27-gauge needles. A small amount of allergen extract (0.02–0.05 mL; 0.02 mL in Hymenoptera to avoid false-positive) is injected into the skin, creating a small bleb 2–3 mm in diameter. Spaces between each injection site should be >2 cm. For patients with a negative prick-puncture test, the concentration of extract for intradermal testing should be between 100- and 1,000-fold more dilute than the concentration used for epicutaneous testing. Variability in test results is due to common errors, which include injecting too deeply, using too much extract, or causing bleeding. Injecting the extract too deeply may hide the response, thereby giving a false-negative result. On the other hand, use of too much extract or bleeding from the prick or puncture may give false-positive results.

Test Controls

Positive and negative test controls are routinely used for the skin test:

Positive Controls

For the **positive control**, histamine at 1 mg/mL for epicutaneous methods and 0.1 mg/ mL for intradermal skin testing is used. A patient must have a positive response to the histamine control to proceed with the skin testing. Mast cell degranulators, such as an opiate, codeine, or morphine sulfate, may also be used as positive controls.

Negative Controls

Diluents used to preserve the allergen extracts are used as **negative controls**. This will help detect any problems with technique, possible skin irritation reaction, or dermatographism.

Indications for Epicutaneous and Intradermal Skin Testing

Skin testing should always begin with epicutaneous testing. If the results of the epicutaneous tests are negative, and there is high clinical suspicion from history, there may be value in proceeding to intradermal skin testing in various situations (Table 8-1). Intradermal skin tests are routinely included in diagnostic testing for allergic bronchopulmonary aspergillosis, penicillin allergy, local anesthetics, and hymenoptera sensitization. **Intradermal testing is never performed for food allergy.**

Interpretation of Skin Test Results

The immediate hypersensitivity reaction can be quantified by measuring the diameter of the wheal and associated erythema (Table 8-2). Wheal size was found to be more specific than erythema size and to correlate better to clinical symptoms. The results should be measured at the peak of the reaction. The peak time for histamine reaction is 8–10 mins, 10–15 mins for mast cell activators such as opiates, and 15–20 mins for allergens. Positive reactions are any wheals that measure >3 mm in diameter.

Praunsnitz-Kustner Test

The Praunsnitz-Kustner test is a passive transfer test and is of historical interest only. This test was the first method by which specific allergic sensitivities were determined before the knowledge of IgE. The serum of a patient with a specific allergy—e.g., to eggs—would be taken and placed on the marked location on the skin of another, nonallergic person. That same spot would be challenged later with the allergen—e.g., the egg

TABLE 8-1. INDICATIONS FOR EPICUTANEOUS AND INTRADERMAL SKIN TESTING

	Epicutaneous	Intradermal
Allergic rhinitis and asthma	Yes	Yes
Food allergy	Yes	Not done
Penicillin allergy	Yes	Yes
Insect venom allergy	Not done	Yes (serial)
Latex allergy	Yes	Not done[a]

[a]No standardized skin test latex reagent is available in the United States. However, one is awaiting FDA approval. Only certain larger medical centers have latex extracts that can be used for skin testing.
From Ownby DR. Diagnostic tests in allergy. In: Lieberman P, Anderson JA, eds. *Allergic diseases diagnosis and treatment*, 2nd ed. Totowa, NJ: Humana Press, 2000;33, with permission.

TABLE 8-2. GRADING SYSTEM FOR SKIN TESTING

Prick test	Intradermal test
1+ erythema <21 mm	3- to 4-mm wheal with erythema
2+ erythema >20 mm	4- to 8-mm wheal without pseudopods
3+ wheal >3 mm	Wheal >8 mm without pseudopods
4+ wheal with pseudopods	Wheal with pseudopods

From Nelson H. Clinical application of immediate skin testing. In Spector SL, ed. *Provocative challenge procedures: background and methodology.* Armonk, NY: Futura, 1989;647, with permission.

protein—and a wheal and flare reaction would be observed. Given the hazards of transmitting bloodborne disease from serum, this test is no longer used.

Set Point Titration

Set point titration is a method developed by Rinkel in which serial dilutions of extract are tested using the intradermal method. Dilutions of allergenic extract increasing in fivefold concentrations are placed and observed for a wheal reaction. A *set point* is defined as the testing dose that initiates an incremental 2-mm increase in the wheal with the fivefold increase in concentration. There is controversy over the scientific validity of this testing method.

IN VITRO TESTING OF IgE

See Table 8-3 for comparison of the advantages of skin testing vs *in vitro* testing.

Total Serum IgE

Total serum IgE can be helpful in identifying persons with high likelihood of atopy but should not be used as a diagnostic or screening test on its own. The test measures total circulating IgE and not the amount of IgE responsible for clinical symptoms. Total serum IgE, therefore, may be elevated in conditions in which the role of IgE is well understood (e.g., asthma; allergic rhinitis; eczema; anaphylaxis from drug, food, or venom; and bronchopulmonary aspergillosis). Difficulty of applying total IgE levels is partly due to their variance with age, especially in the pediatric population, and the considerable overlap between normal and atopic individuals. This range of overlap is anywhere from 20 to 180 IU/mL of total IgE. Thus, minor elevated levels of IgE will not be helpful. Usually, levels that are >1,800 IU/mL indicate a likely diagnosis of

TABLE 8-3. COMPARATIVE ADVANTAGES OF SKIN TESTING VS *IN VITRO* TESTING FOR DIAGNOSIS OF ALLERGY

Advantages of skin tests	Advantages of *in vitro* tests
High sensitivity	No risk of anaphylaxis
Results available in minutes	Medications do not affect results
Greater selection of allergen	Not dependent on skin condition
Cheaper than *in vitro* tests	Convenient for patients afraid of needles
Minimal equipment needed	Perceived by patients as more scientific

atopy, whereas levels <20 IU/mL make diagnosis of atopy unlikely. Moreover, it is important to rule out other causes of elevated total IgE levels.

Other Conditions with Increased Total IgE

- Tobacco use
- Alcoholism
- Parasitic infection
- HIV
- IgE multiple myeloma
- Wiskott-Aldrich syndrome
- Job syndrome
- Churg-Strauss vasculitis
- Hyper-IgE syndrome
- Pemphigoid
- Hodgkin's disease
- Omenn's syndrome
- Severe burns

Antigen-Specific IgE

In contrast to total serum IgE, antigen-specific IgE is of great clinical importance. The most widely used procedure is the **RAST**, which was one of the first tests developed to detect antigen-specific IgE. More sophisticated methods, such as the ELISA, which uses enzymatic reaction instead of the radiolabeled IgE immunoglobulins, are available, but all of the tests that detect antigen-specific IgE are collectively referred to as *radioallergosorbant tests*.

All use the basic principle of immunoabsorption. First, the antigen in question is bound to a solid phase (e.g., a paper disk, cellulose sponge, or plastic microtiter well plate). Then, a patient's serum is incubated with the solid phase. After washing, a labeled anti–human IgE is incubated with the solid phase. After another washing, the amount of labeled anti-IgE is measured and reported either in absolute IgE units or as a class score. A class score of 0 is negative, scores in the range 0–1 are considered indeterminate, and any score >2 is considered positive and should be correlated with clinical history.

DIAGNOSTIC TESTING FOR ALLERGIC CONTACT DERMATITIS

The **patch skin test** is the most useful tool in diagnosis of allergic contact dermatitis. Unlike epicutaneous and intradermal skin testing, patch testing is a measure of a **delayed hypersensitivity** reaction. The test artificially attempts to reproduce the clinical symptoms of the patient and helps to determine provocative antigens. However, it has limitations in that the sensitivity and specificity are only 70%, even when performed by the most experienced clinicians.

Method

Preparation of the Patient

Antihistamines are not contraindicated. Topical corticosteroids should not be applied to the patch test site for several days before testing. Oral corticosteroids should ideally be discontinued for 1 wk before testing. Patch testing may be performed with reasonable sensitivity in chronic users of steroids when the dose is ≤15 mg/day.

1. First, it is important to determine that the area of skin to be tested is without irritation or inflammation.
2. Small amounts of diluted testing materials are placed on small aluminum disks and are placed on the patient's back, under nonocclusive dressing with hypoaller-

genic tape. Each test material's concentration should be sufficiently dilute to minimize the chance of an irritant reaction. Again, clinical history should narrow the number of suspected antigens. Standard testing kits are also available commercially.

3. For the 2 days after placement of the patch tests (or until the test sites are graded), the patient should not bathe, shower, or participate in strenuous activities.

4. The patient returns in 48–72 hrs for removal of the disks and grading of the test areas. The patient should return for a late reading 4–5 days after original application. The late reading will increase sensitivity, because some reactions may not be evident at the first reading.

Allergen Panels

Only 23 commercially prepared allergens are FDA-approved in the United States. There are several patch test kits containing these allergens; one is described in Table 8-4 (note

TABLE 8-4. PANEL OF ALLERGENS IN T.R.U.E. TEST

Allergen	Environmental occurrences
Nickel sulfate	Jewelry, metal
Wool alcohols (lanolin)	Cosmetics, soaps, topical medications
Neomycin sulfate	Topical antibiotics
Potassium dichromate	Cement, cutting oils
Caine mix	Topical anesthetics
Fragrance mix	Toiletries, scented household products
Colophony	Cosmetics, adhesives
Paraben mix	Preservative in topical formulations and foods
Negative control	—
Balsam of Peru	Foods, cosmetics
Ethylenediamine dihydrochloride	Topical medicines, industrial solvents
Cobalt dichloride	Metal-plated objects, paints
p-*tert*-Butylphenol formaldehyde resin	Waterproof glues, bonded leather
Epoxy resin	Two-part adhesives, paints
Carba mix	Rubber products, glues for leather, vinyl
Black rubber mix	All black rubber products, some hair dyes
Cl + Me-isothiazolinone	Cosmetics, topical medicines
Quaternium-15	Preservative in cosmetics, household cleaners
Mercaptobenzothiazole	Rubber products, adhesives
p-Phenylenediamine	Hair dyes, dyed textiles
Formaldehyde	Fabric finishes, plastics, synthetic resins
Mercapto mix	Rubber products, glues for leather/plastics
Thimerosal	Preservative in contact lens solutions and injectable drugs
Thiuram mix	Rubber products, adhesives

Modified from http://www.truetest.com/physician/comp.htm. See the website for specific information, including concentrations of each allergen and cross-reactivity.

that one component is a negative control). The thiuram mix may be helpful in identifying sensitivity to thiuram accelerators used in manufacturing latex products.

Precautions

The application of the patch test may itself sensitize the patient or cause a flare-up in an already-sensitized patient. Patients should be instructed to remove any patch that is causing severe irritation. Repeated patch testing should be avoided. Standardized concentrations of test material should be used to avoid an inflammatory reaction, and thus a false-positive result.

Grading

Grades 1+ and above are positive.

- 0 (negative): no detectable change in appearance of skin
- 1+: erythema with edema covering at least $1/2$ of test area
- 2+: erythema and edema plus papules
- 3+: vesicles and bullae plus erythema, edema, and papules

False-Positive and False-Negative Results

False-positive test results may be due to the following: (a) skin may be hypersensitive to one of the antigens, and, therefore, the entire back can become inflamed; and (b) irritation due to factors other than antigen (e.g., the tape used).

False-negative test results may be due to the following: (a) concentration of antigen was too low, (b) technical errors in applying the antigen patches, and (c) late reading at 3–7 days not performed.

Clinical Application of Test Results

It is important to remember that a positive patch skin test result does not mean diagnosis of causative agent for contact dermatitis. The antigen could be a secondary aggravating factor. Thus, positive test results should be correlated with clinical history, and, when possible, the patient should avoid the antigens that caused a positive reaction.

KEY POINTS

- Diagnostic testing is helpful in confirming allergic basis for disease and in guiding treatment when used in conjunction with a careful history and physical.
- Medications that can interfere with skin testing should be discontinued for the appropriate length of time.
- Total serum IgE alone should not be used as a diagnostic or screening tool.
- Skin testing should be deferred in patients who have had a recent anaphylactic reaction.
- Patch skin testing is most helpful in diagnosis of allergic contact dermatitis and measures delayed hypersensitivity to specific allergens.

SUGGESTED READING

Bousquet J, Michel F-B. Diagnostic tests. In: Korenblat PE, Wedner HJ, eds. *Allergy: theory and practice*, 2nd ed. Philadelphia: WB Saunders, 1992;143–163.

Demoly P, Michel F-B, Bosquet J. In vivo methods for study of allergy skin tests, techniques, and interpretation. In: Middleton E Jr, ed. *Allergy: principles and practice*, 5th ed. St. Louis: Mosby–Year Book, 1998;430–439.

Merrett TG. Quantification of IgE both as total immunoglobulin and as allergen-specific antibody. In: Kay AB, ed. *Allergy and allergic diseases*, vol 2. Boston: Blackwell Science, 1997;1012–1033.

Nelson H. Clinical application of immediate skin testing. In: Spector SL, ed. *Provocative challenge procedures: background and methodology*. New York: Futura, 1989;639–665.

Ownby DR. Diagnostic tests in allergy. In: Lieberman P, Anderson JA, eds. *Allergic diseases diagnosis and treatment*, 2nd ed. Totowa, NJ: Humana, 2000;29–39.

Urticaria and Angioedema

Elizabeth C. Friedman

INTRODUCTION

As much as 15–20% of the U.S. population will experience urticaria or angioedema at some time in their life. Although urticaria is often mild and self-limited, it may become chronic or occur as a component of potentially life-threatening anaphylaxis. Chronic idiopathic urticaria (CIU) is common, affecting 0.1% of the population with an economic and social burden comparable to that seen with severe coronary artery disease. Although lesions of urticaria/angioedema are histologically the same regardless of the cause, differences in etiology and therapy warrant the classification into acute and chronic syndromes.

Definition

Urticaria consists of raised, erythematous areas of edema that involve only the superficial dermis of the skin. The lesions are usually pruritic and may develop rapidly. **Any single lesion does not ordinarily last >24 hrs.** In contrast, **angioedema** extends into the deep dermis or subcutaneous tissue and often affects areas of loose connective tissue, such as the face. Angioedema may be uncomfortable or painful rather than pruritic, especially when the viscera are involved, and can last for several days. Angioedema involving a patient's larynx can threaten the airway and lead to asphyxiation.

Classification

The syndrome is defined as **acute** if the lesions are of **<6 wks'** duration. Often, the cause is obvious and self-limited. The most common causes of acute urticaria are reactions to foods and drugs.

Chronic urticaria/angioedema has lesions that have lasted **>6 wks**. The syndrome lasts an average of 3–5 yrs, with 20% of patients still symptomatic at 20 yrs. The syndrome is frustrating to patient and clinician alike in that a search for an exogenous cause is futile in the majority of patients. However, in recent years, it has been demonstrated that many patients with CIU exhibit autoantibodies directed against the high-affinity IgE receptor (see Autoimmune Chronic Urticaria). In addition to autoimmune urticaria, several physical urticarial syndromes are important to define, because once diagnosed, no further workup is necessary (see Physical Urticaria Syndromes).

CAUSES

Pathophysiology

Histamine is the principal mediator of urticaria and angioedema; however, other mediators, such as prostaglandin D_2, leukotrienes C and D, platelet activating factor, and components of the complement and coagulation cascades, can be involved. This complexity explains why antihistamines sometimes may not be completely effective. The **mast cell** is the major effector in all forms of urticaria and angioedema, although other cells, such as basophils, are also involved. Urticaria and angioedema may result from direct mast cell stimulation (as in reactions to opiate drugs), IgE-mediated hypersensitivity, or components of the complement or arachidonic acid pathways. The lesions may also be idiopathic. They infrequently occur in association with several systemic diseases (see History).

Differential Diagnosis

- **Erythema multiforme minor:** Lesions persist rather than wax/wane. Lesions are usually preceded by a prodrome of constitutional symptoms.
- **Bullous pemphigoid and dermatitis herpetiformis:** Initial presentation may be similar but the formation of bullae rules out urticaria.
- **Mastocytosis:** History is often helpful. Characteristic lesions of urticaria pigmentosa, mastocytoma, and telangiectasia eruptive macularis perstans (TEMP) (see Chap. 19, Mastocytosis).

PRESENTATION

History

A detailed history and review of systems are far more likely to reveal the cause of urticaria than almost any diagnostic test and should include the following:

- **Drug reactions:** List all current and recent prescription and over-the-counter medications and herbal supplements. The most common drugs causing hives are **antibiotics** and **opiate analgesics**. ACE inhibitors, nonselective beta-blockers, ASA, and NSAIDs may cause or exacerbate urticaria and/or angioedema. There are sporadic cases of specific NSAIDs causing urticaria, but in general, all NSAIDs cross-react.
- **Food ingestions:** Fish, milk, eggs, wheat, soy, nuts, and peanuts are the most common foods causing urticaria, although a person may develop an allergy to potentially any food (see Chap. 16, Food Allergy and Other Adverse Food Reactions).
- Physical stimuli: related to lesions (see Physical Urticaria Syndromes).
- Evidence of infection: Viral hepatitis, mononucleosis, fungal infections, helminthes (usually accompanied by high eosinophilia) have all been associated with urticaria. The association between *Helicobacter pylori* infection and urticaria remains controversial.
- Aeroallergen: Rarely, patients with seasonal allergies experience urticaria/angioedema during episodes of high exposure.
- **Recent sting or insect bite:** History is usually obvious (see Chap. 15, Insect Allergy).
- **Food additives:** Rare causes of urticaria/angioedema, but reactions to some food additives and dyes have been reported (see Chap. 16, Food Allergy and Other Adverse Food Reactions).
- Family history of similar lesions? Consider hereditary angioedema or a familial urticarial syndrome (see Hereditary Angioedema or Familial Urticarial Syndrome).
- **Review of systems** for collagen vascular disease, hepatic disease, autoimmune thyroiditis, lymphoproliferative disorders, and malignancy. The latter two are associated with acquired C1 inhibitor deficiency.

Physical Urticaria Syndromes

- **Cold urticaria:** Seen on cold, exposed areas of skin. Test with an ice cube on forearm for 3 mins; lesions seen on re-warming. Fatalities have been reported from hypotension occurring while swimming. Secondary acquired cold urticaria is related to cryoglobulins resulting from systemic disease (hepatitis B or C) or lymphoreticular malignancy. Treatment is directed at any underlying disorder plus antihistamines.
- **Cholinergic (heat) urticaria:** Related to elevated core temperature from exercise, a hot shower, or emotional stress; test by running vigorously in place for 10 mins. **Lesions are typically tiny and diffuse.** A very common physical urticaria, occurring

in approximately 15% of the population. Severe forms may progress to angioedema and syncope although lesions usually resolve if the patient "cools off." Treatment consists of antihistamines.

- **Dermographism:** Literally "skin writing," another common form of physical urticaria. Effects approximately 4% of the population. Briskly stroke skin with tongue blade or fingernail. Note linear lesions from excoriation on exam. May confound ability to read allergen skin tests. Lesions are transitory and respond to suppression with antihistamines.
- **Pressure urticaria/angioedema:** Unlike other physical urticaria, lesions appear 4–6 hrs after the stimulus of pressure. Test with 15-lb weight in a sling over forearm. Mediators are thought to be similar to late-phase reactants rather than histamine. Thus, this disorder is poorly responsive to antihistamines; systemic steroids may be needed to control severely afflicted patients.
- **Vibratory urticaria.** Rare disorder. Test by holding patient's forearm on a lab vortex for 4 mins.
- **Solar urticaria:** History usually establishes the diagnosis. Very rare disorder. Different categories depending on wavelength of light-producing symptoms. One type is synonymous with erythropoietic protoporphyria, and patients with this disorder should have serum protoporphyrin checked.
- **Exercise-induced anaphylaxis:** Different from cholinergic urticaria in that it is **not related to core body temperature**. Lesions are typically urticarial and progress to anaphylaxis. In some patients, the ingestion of a specific food before exercise is necessary to trigger the reaction, although eating before exercise in general will worsen symptoms in most patients. **Patients should carry epinephrine and antihistamines.**
- **Aquagenic urticaria:** Exceedingly rare. Patients react to a wet compress regardless of its temperature.

Familial Urticaria/Angioedema Syndromes

Most of the familial urticaria/angioedema syndromes, such as familial cold urticaria, hereditary vibratory angioedema, and C3b inactivator deficiency, are quite rare and are mentioned for completeness. Only the more common ones are discussed in detail here.

Hereditary Angioedema

The name of the disorder is somewhat problematic, because although the majority of patients possess an **autosomal dominant heredity**, spontaneous mutations cause the disorder in 15–25% of patients. It is caused by **absence or dysfunction of C1 esterase inhibitor** and is characterized by periodic attacks of angioedema that are often, but not always, triggered by trauma (i.e., dental surgery). **Onset of angioedema** is usually at puberty, although some patients experience attacks of abdominal pain with guarding in the absence of leukocytosis and fever as children. These symptoms represent angioedema of the viscera.

DIAGNOSIS. Diagnosis is made by an initial screening C4 level that is always low and can drop to undetectable levels during an attack. If the C4 level is low, obtain a C1 inhibitor level. In approximately 15–20% of patients, the level is normal, but the protein is not functional, and a functional assay must be performed.

TREATMENT

Acute Attacks.   Provide supportive care in acute attacks. Isolated limb swelling can be observed. Laryngeal swelling may lead to **asphyxiation** and is the **leading cause of mortality and morbidity** in patients with this disorder. Intubation must be considered electively before laryngeal swelling makes this difficult or impossible. Appropriate personnel and equipment for a tracheotomy should be available. Epinephrine has often been used for attacks, but there are no studies to support its efficacy. The pain of severe swelling has historically been managed with meperidine (Demerol). **Fluid resuscitation** may be necessary secondary to third spacing. A C1 inhibitor cryoprecipitate will rapidly control symptoms; however, it is not available in the United States. **Debate exists regarding the use of fresh frozen plasma** during an acute attack, as this has been seen to worsen symptoms in a few patients (see Prophylaxis).

Long-Term Therapy. Synthetic androgenic steroids (danazol [Danocrine] or stanozolol [Winstrol]) have attenuated virilizing side effects and can improve symptoms in patients with frequent occurrences. However, side effects do still occur. Counseling to women of childbearing age is necessary because of interference with gonadal development. Fibrinolytic agents (such as ε-aminocaproic acid) have also been shown to ameliorate symptoms. Unfortunately, this therapy also carries the risk of numerous side effects. Decision for therapy must be made on an individual basis.

Prophylaxis. The use of agents for allergic urticaria and corticosteroids are of little value. Androgens are also ineffective in the acute setting but may be given 4–5 days before scheduled surgery. Other agents that may be used prophylactically are antifibrinolytics and fresh frozen plasma.

Acquired Angioedema

Findings for acquired angioedema are similar to those for hereditary angioedema. Symptoms are the result of a **C1q autoantibody**. A low C1q level combined with low C1 inhibitor and C4 levels warrants an investigation for an occult malignancy, because this disorder is associated with lymphoproliferative disorders. It is also rarely associated with connective tissue disease.

Urticarial Vasculitis

Exam usually reveals lesions in **dependent areas**. Other signs of vasculitis, such as petechiae and palpable purpura, are often evident. Lesions tend to **last >24 hrs** and be more **painful** than pruritic. **A punch biopsy is necessary to make the diagnosis** and will show necrotizing vasculitis. Lesions are thought to be due to immune complex–mediated inflammation. Urticarial vasculitis is associated with numerous conditions, including collagen vascular disease, chronic hepatitis, Lyme disease, myelomas, and cryoglobulinemias, as well as others.

Autoimmune Chronic Urticaria

Studies have shown a subset of patients with CIU have autoantibodies directed against the high-affinity IgE receptor. In some patients, autologous skin testing (using the patient's serum) is positive. However, this is not diagnostic, as these autoantibodies can be seen in other disease states and in some normal patients. Some success has been achieved with the use of dapsone and cyclosporine, the latter requiring initial monitoring of serum levels and renal function.

Physical Exam

Note pattern of lesions if one exists. A thorough exam is required to detect any of the underlying conditions described above.

MANAGEMENT

Diagnosis

The history usually elicits a cause or underlying condition; thus, the workup should be directed specifically. Resist the shotgun approach to obtaining labs. Occasionally, it is necessary to challenge the patient with a suspected agent. See Chap. 14, Drug Allergy and Desensitization, and Chap. 16, Food Allergy and Other Adverse Food Reactions, for specifics regarding drug and food testing. These tests should only be performed by physicians trained to interpret the results. If no cause is apparent, consider:

- **Lab studies:** CBC, urinalysis, sedimentation rate, liver function tests, antithyroid antibodies.

- Removal of **exacerbating agents** such as NSAIDs, opiates, and alcohol; may aid in the diagnosis.
- **Elimination diet:** Some advocate an elimination diet of rice, lamb, and water when a food is suspected as the cause. New foods are introduced one at a time as they are tolerated. Compliance is the main hurdle with this endeavor. **Food diaries** can help direct specific IgE tests.

Treatment

Choice of treatment depends on the etiology of the lesions. It may involve avoidance (as in NSAIDs or opiates), specific therapy (some physical urticarias respond to antihistamines), or treatment of an underlying condition (such as thyroid replacement for autoimmune thyroiditis).

In the presence of systemic symptoms suggesting anaphylaxis, **epinephrine** (0.3–0.5 mL 1:1,000 SC) should be rapidly administered. **Patients should be given an injectable form of epinephrine** and instructed in its use regardless of whether the cause of these symptoms has been determined. The EpiPen does not require a patient to self-administer a hypodermic needle, is simply pressed against one of the extremities, and comes in pediatric and adult strengths (see Chap. 13, Anaphylaxis).

Second-generation antihistamines are either nonsedating (fexofenadine [Allegra], loratadine [Claritin], or desloratadine [Clarinex]) or low sedating (cetirizine [Zyrtec]). They are usually well tolerated and given daily can often control symptoms until they remit. First-generation antihistamines, such as diphenhydramine (Benadryl) and cyproheptadine (Periactin), can also be effective, but excess sedation and anticholinergic side effects often limit their use. Patients may report they do not feel sedated, but slowed reaction times have been reported even at standard doses.

H_2-blocking antihistamines can be added if symptoms are not controlled.

If pruritus is not controlled with traditional antihistamines, **doxepin** (Sinequan) can be added, because it acts as a more potent antihistamine than H_1 blockers. The typical dose is 10 mg at bedtime. Doxepin can be very sedating; thus, the same caution regarding daytime somnolence and slowed reaction times applies.

A short burst of **prednisone** (Deltasone) can often eradicate symptoms but has numerous, well-documented side effects. Therefore, steroids should be used in severe cases or in cases refractory to antihistamines. The dose and course should be high enough and long enough to control symptoms. Tapering steroids is not necessary to prevent adrenal suppression for courses shorter than 3 wks but can be helpful to determine if symptoms have remitted and to achieve the lowest effective dose. Typical doses are 40–60 mg/day for severe exacerbations. Patients should be adequately counseled regarding side effects associated with steroids (irritability/euphoria, water retention, glucose intolerance, appetite stimulation, and sleep disturbance).

KEY POINTS

- If an exogenous cause is to be found, it will be discovered by taking a good history.
- In chronic urticaria, an exogenous cause is rarely found. Avoid the shotgun approach to labs, but look for a systemic disease.
- Any single urticarial lesion usually lasts no longer than 24 hrs. If otherwise, consider urticarial vasculitis or an alternative diagnosis.
- Low-sedating or nonsedating antihistamines can be effective for pruritis, making somnolence from first-generation antihistamines unnecessary. However, when sleep is disrupted, diphenhydramine (Benadryl) or doxepin (Sinequan) may be helpful.

SUGGESTED READING

Grattan CH, O'Donnell BF, Francis DM, et al. Randomized double-blind study of cyclosporin in chronic 'idiopathic' urticaria. *Br J Dermatol* 2000;143(2):365–372.
Greaves M. Chronic urticaria. *J Allergy Clin Immunol* 2000;105(4):664–672.

Kaplan AP. Urticaria and angioedema. In: Middleton E, ed. *Allergy: principles and practice*, 5th ed. St. Louis: Mosby, 1998;1104–1122.

Tharp MD. Chronic urticaria: pathophysiology and treatment approaches. *J Allergy Clin Immunol* 1996;98(6).

The diagnosis and management of urticaria: a practice parameter part I: acute urticaria/angioedema part II: chronic urticaria/angioedema. Joint Task Force on Practice Parameters. *Ann Allergy Asthma Immunol* 2000;85(6):521–544.

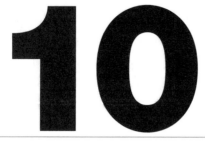

Atopic Dermatitis

Khaled M. Abdel-Hamid

INTRODUCTION

Definition

Atopic dermatitis (AD) is a chronic, relapsing, and intensely pruritic skin disease. It has been previously known as *atopic eczema, neurodermatitis*, and *prurigo Besnier*. The distribution of the skin lesions and the atopic background of the patient tend to suggest the diagnosis more than the appearance of the lesions themselves.

Epidemiology

The prevalence of AD in the general population has been estimated to be 0.7–2% and is similar in men and women. Higher prevalence of 4–5% is observed in children. Recent studies have suggested that prevalence of AD has been increasing over the last 30 yrs, with recent estimates as high as 8–10% in children. This increase is not unique to AD and is paralleled by increases in the prevalence of other atopic diseases, such as allergic rhinitis and bronchial asthma.

CAUSES

Pathophysiology

Increased Immunoglobulin E

Over 80% of AD patients have elevated serum IgE. The elevation is frequently proportional to the extent, severity, and level of disease activity. Occasionally, the levels reach >1,500 IU (1 IU = 2.4 ng/mL). IgE levels tend to decline after periods of disease inactivity and in well-controlled AD patients. Normal IgE level does not, however, rule out AD. The exact role of increased IgE in the pathogenesis of AD is not clear. However, skin prick tests (SPTs) and RASTs are commonly used to screen for trigger allergens, such as foods, dander, mites, and pollens, with the aim of eliminating possible triggers. Antigen-specific IgE may contribute to the pathogenesis of AD via a delayed late-phase reaction rather than an immediate early-phase reaction such as those observed in urticaria and allergic rhinitis.

Specific Allergens

Specific allergens can be identified using skin tests and/or *in vitro* testing in AD patients. The significance of these allergens in the pathogenesis, maintenance, and aggravation of AD is not always clear. In most AD patients, positive SPT or RAST tests simply reflect the patients' atopic background and not a role for the specific allergen(s) in disease activity. However, using elimination diets and double-blind, placebo-controlled food challenges (DBPCFCs), 30% of children with AD show disease exacerbation in response to specific food challenges (commonly egg, milk, wheat, soy, or nuts). These patients outgrow their food allergies as they outgrow their AD. In adults, the association between food allergens and disease activity is usually lacking.

In some adults and children, dust mites, animal danders, and, in rare cases, other aeroallergens have been identified as triggers for AD. Seasonal exacerbation of AD suggests reaction to pollen components.

Impaired Cutaneous Lymphocyte Function

Impaired cutaneous lymphocyte function has been reported in AD patients. This is characterized by reduced delayed hypersensitivity skin responses as well as decreased lymphocyte responses to mitogens *in vitro*. The number of $CD8^+$ lymphocytes is also reduced, providing a potential mechanism for increased serum IgE. The prevalence of **cutaneous (but not systemic)** viral infections, such as herpes simplex, molluscum contagiosum, and skin warts, is **higher** in AD, a potential clinical correlate to the impaired cutaneous lymphocyte hypothesis.

Staphylococcus aureus *or Dermatophyte Skin Colonization*

Staphylococcus aureus or dermatophyte skin colonization may be a contributing factor to the pathogenesis of AD. Nine out of ten patients with AD have skin lesions colonized with *S. aureus*. Half of these patients have demonstrable IgE against staphylococcal exotoxins (e.g., toxic shock syndrome toxin-1, enterotoxins A and B). Similarly, dermatophyte infection (especially with *Pityrosporum*) with positive antifungal SPTs and RASTs can be detected in nearly half of the older children and adults with recalcitrant head, neck, and upper body AD. The mechanism underlying the association between AD and these infections is not clear, although IgE-mediated and staphylococcal superantigen mechanisms have been entertained [1].

Skin Hyperirritability

Skin hyperirritability with increased numbers of mast cells and skin histamine content has also been reported in AD. It is unclear whether this is a primary or a secondary phenomenon. Skin hyperirritability manifests itself as an exacerbation of skin lesions in response to large number of environmental triggers in a non–immune-mediated fashion. These triggers include detergents, certain fabrics (wool and acrylic), dust, extreme temperature and humidity, emotional stress, perfumes, and so forth.

Differential Diagnosis

Seborrheic dermatitis, contact dermatitis, dermatophytosis, pompholyx, lichen simplex chronicum, and drug eruptions.
    In children:

- Psoriasis, scabies, and diaper rash need to be ruled out.
- Less commonly, AD-like skin disease can be a manifestation of immune deficiency (e.g., ataxia telangiectasia, Wiskott-Aldrich syndrome, X-linked agammaglobulinemia, and hyper-IgE syndrome).
- Skin manifestations of metabolic disorder, such as phenylketonuria, or nutritional deficiencies associated with malabsorption syndromes can be confused with AD skin eruptions as well.

    In adults, especially with **late onset or recalcitrant** disease, Sézary syndrome and cutaneous T-cell **lymphomas must be considered**.

Natural History

50% of the patients who develop AD show manifestations of the disease by 12 mos of age, and frequently the disease is evident by the second month of life. By 5 yrs, 90% of the patients have established disease. Although AD can develop at any age, new-onset dermatitis presenting in adulthood is unlikely to be AD.
    90% of children with AD at 5 yrs outgrow their disease by 15 yrs. However, some patients continue to suffer from AD throughout life. The disease course can be of chronic or relapsing nature. Despite the atopic nature of the disease, it is sometimes

difficult to find strong clinical correlation between allergen exposure and disease severity or activity. In other cases, the association is more pronounced (e.g., precipitation of AD after the introduction of a new food into a child's diet).

PRESENTATION

Risk Factors

Risk factors for severe and chronic AD include disease onset before 12 mos of age, severe disease in childhood, and atopic background (positive family history, coincident allergic rhinitis and/or asthma). Females also have higher propensity for severe and chronic AD.

Clinical Presentation

AD has been described as the **itching that erupts, not the eruption that itches** [2]. This statement emphasizes the temporal, and possibly causal, relationship between the two salient features of AD. Thus, intense itching is commonly the primary symptom, with skin lesions appearing where the mechanical irritation (scratching) takes place. Once skin lesions are established, nonspecific irritants tend to maintain the vicious cycle (**itch → scratch → skin hyperirritability → itch**).

Understanding this mechanism has important therapeutic implications and highlights the importance of patient education and managing psychosocial stresses. It also helps explain the efficacy of sedating histamine antagonists, the importance of appropriate skin hygiene, and the need for nonspecific trigger control. However, this should not lead to underestimating the significance of allergic triggers, such as foods, in many pediatric patients.

Physical Findings

Distribution of the skin lesions tends to follow an age-dependent pattern that is unique to AD and is frequently the main clue to the diagnosis.

- In **infants and young children**, the lesions usually start on the scalp, forehead, and cheeks. Later, the disease spreads to the trunk and extremities, with predilection for the extensor surfaces. **The diaper region is characteristically spared.**
- In **older children** (2–11 yrs), AD tends to affect the flexural areas of extremities (antecubital and popliteal fossae, anterior of wrists and ankles) as well as the perioral region and the neck. This pattern also persists in adolescents and adults, with additional involvement of the upper trunk.
- In some patients, the disease is more aggressive, with larger areas of the body involved. In other cases, especially in young women, **hand eczema** may be the only manifestation of the disease.

Acute lesions are more common in infants and young children. The skin may show oozing **erythematous patches, papules, small vesicles, and scales**. Occasionally, yellow, crusty discharge may be present, suggesting coexistence of bacterial infection (S. aureus). Nonlesional skin may be dry with fine sandpaper-like texture.

Chronic lesions are more common as the course of the disease advances. These are **thick lichenified skin patches with fissuring and fibrotic papules**. There are also areas of hypo- and hyperpigmentation consistent with the chronic inflammatory nature of the disease. The affected skin is generally dry with many scratch marks, ulcers, and denuded areas secondary to trauma and infections (impetigo). In many patients, isolated hand lesions (hand eczema) and, less frequently, perioral skin changes (cheilitis) may be observed.

Less common findings include other stigmata of atopic diseases (Dennie's line, allergic shiners), keratoconus, anterior subcapsular cataract (in a small number of adults after 5–10 yrs of severe AD), hyperkeratosis pilaris (chicken-skin texture of lateral skin of extremities and buttocks), pityriasis alba (round hypopigmented macules over face, extremities and upper trunk), ichthyosis, and **white dermatographism** (delayed blanching of **lesional and nonlesional skin** after light stroking, pressure, or exposure to cold).

AD runs a chronic course, with periods of exacerbation and remission. Triggers include the following:

- Certain **foods**, via an immune mechanism, may exacerbate the disease in children but rarely do so in adults. **Egg is the most commonly reported offender.** Less common food triggers include milk, wheat, soy, nuts, and fish. These foods were shown in DBPCFCs to contribute to AD disease activity in one-third of children with AD.
- Some **aeroallergens** were also found to contribute to AD. Strong evidence supports a role for dust mites and animal dander, whereas less convincing evidence implicates *Alternaria* and cockroach allergens.
- **Psychosocial** factors, such as stress and sleep deprivation, can trigger AD flares.
- Nonspecific **skin irritants**, such as wool and synthetic fiber fabric, hot humid weather, cold dry weather, excess sun exposure, scented laundry detergents, laundry bleach, harsh soaps, and perfumes, can trigger AD flares. Certain foods may aggravate skin condition **on contact**, secondary to their strong physical properties (e.g., acidic citrus fruits), and **are not immune mediated.**

MANAGEMENT

Diagnosis

Major diagnostic criteria for AD include chronic or relapsing intense pruritus, early age of onset, atopic background (family history or co-existing allergic rhinitis or bronchial asthma), and age-appropriate skin rash (see Physical Findings).

Workup

Skin Testing
Skin testing can be useful in identifying allergens for the purpose of environmental control measures. These measures are usually more useful for the control of atopic comorbidity such as allergic rhinitis (and possibly bronchial asthma) than for AD. Skin tests have excellent negative predictive value and thus can help avoid unnecessary avoidance measures (e.g., extreme elimination diets resulting in malnutrition). These tests, however, do not have good positive predictive value, and thus in children with positive food SPTs, a positive DBPCFC is frequently necessary before recommending the elimination of these foods from diet.

Blood Tests
Lab tests are of limited value in diagnosis and management of AD. RASTs are less sensitive than skin tests for detection of antigen-specific IgE but may occasionally be necessary if skin tests are not feasible or contraindicated (e.g., diffuse skin lesions or strong history of food-induced anaphylaxis). Total IgE is frequently elevated (but may be normal), and eosinophilia may be present. Neither finding is specific for AD.

Treatment

The pillars of effective AD treatment are skin hydration, topical corticosteroids, and trigger avoidance. Education is crucial for effective participation of patients in their own care.

Education
AD is a potentially chronic and difficult to manage disease with unpleasant and stressful symptoms (pruritus and skin lesions). Poor sleep, frequent aggravations by many

normal daily activities, and disfiguring facial and hand lesions all contribute to emotional stress in patients and their families. The natural history of AD, the value of skin hydration and environmental control, and the importance of itch-scratch cycle control should be the initial objectives of patient education. Adequate education is essential for the formation of a good therapeutic alliance.

Environmental and Trigger Control

- Avoid extreme temperatures and humidity.
- Use dust mite control measures: dust mite covers on pillows and mattresses, wash bedding in hot water (130°F) weekly, and maintain relative humidity <50%.
- Avoid contact with animal dander.
- Avoid tight, nonbreathing clothes and excessive exposure to sunlight without protective creams.
- Avoid wool, acrylic, and coarse fabrics. Cotton is the preferred fabric for clothes.

Skin Care and Hydration

- Use unscented laundry detergents without bleach. Double rinsing is recommended.
- Avoid skin exposure to solvents and irritating vapors.
- Maintain skin hydration by **bathing with tepid water** (30 mins once or twice daily, depending on severity of disease), using oatmeal or baking soda bath and unscented mild soaps (e.g., Neutrogena, Dove, Basis). Showering is usually not adequate for good skin hydration. Avoid excessive or vigorous toweling.
- Apply **emollients** such as Eucerin, Nutraderm, Aquaphor, or petroleum jelly generously within 3 mins after bathing to **"lock in" skin moisture**.
- **Trim nails short** to minimize skin trauma. Wearing **gloves and socks** during sleep helps limit scratching.
- Wet dressing or water-soaked pajamas worn under waterproof tracksuits maximize skin hydration in chronic resistant AD. Skin hydration is soothing, reduces itch and bacterial colonization, and even improves topical corticosteroid skin penetration.

Medications

CORTICOSTEROIDS. **Topical steroids** are the mainstays of AD antiinflammatory treatment. For mild cases, a low-potency steroid ointment or cream (hydrocortisone [Cortef, Hydrocortone] 1–2.5%, bid/qid) may be adequate. Medium-potency steroids (mometasone furoate [Elocon] 0.1% qd or triamcinolone [Aristocort, Kenalog, Triacet] 0.025–0.1% tid/qid) are required for more severe forms of the disease.

Please note that recent clinical trials suggest that moderate and severe AD may initially be treated with the **topical immunosupressants** tacrolimus (Protopic) and pimecrolimus (Elidel) instead of higher-potency topical steroids for several months, then maintaining disease control using lower potency topical steroids if necessary.

Ointments are more efficacious than creams and should be used whenever possible. Creams may be adequate for milder forms of AD. Topical steroids can be applied over emollients used to maintain skin hydration.

Localized flares may be treated with high-potency topical steroids, such as clobetasol propionate (Clobevate, Cormax, Embeline E, Olux, Temovate) (0.05% bid) or halobetasol [Ultravate] (0.05% bid/tid), for 10–14 days followed by medium-potency topical steroids. High-potency steroids should be used sparingly and never on the face. If used for longer periods, the adrenal cortex may be suppressed, and tapering of the topical steroid is necessary.

High-potency corticosteroids should never be used on the face, intertriginous areas, or genitals. These areas should be treated with low-potency topical steroids only (e.g., hydrocortisone 1%).

Systemic corticosteroids have no place in the long-term treatment of AD. Widespread severe flares may require moderate doses of prednisone (Deltasone, Liquid Pred, Meticorten, Orasone, Prednicen-M, Sterapred) (40–60 mg/day), tapered by 20 mg/day every 4–5 days, with adequate topical coverage to follow. Abrupt interruption of systemic corticosteroid treatment may be associated with an exacerbation of dermatitis. **A recurrent need for systemic steroids is an indication for referral to a specialist** to consider alternative therapies.

ANTIHISTAMINES. H_1-histamine receptor blockers do not alter the course of the disease but are used for their antipruritic effect. Sedating antihistamines can be used at divided doses or as bedtime dose to control pruritus and improve sleep. **The combined antipruritic/sedating effect probably underlies the higher efficacy of sedating antihistamines compared to their more expensive, nonsedating counterparts.** High doses of antihistamines are frequently needed (e.g., diphenhydramine [Benadryl, Benylin] to a maximum 400 mg/day; hydroxyzine (Atarax, Rezine, Vistaril) up to 100 mg/day in divided doses).

Nonsedating second-generation antihistamines have no therapeutic advantage over sedating antihistamines. However, for some patients, a **combination of daytime nonsedating antihistamine (cetirizine [Zyrtec], loratadine [Claritin], or fexofenadine [Allegra]) and bedtime sedating antihistamine (diphenhydramine or hydroxyzine)** may provide symptomatic control without the daytime sedation that may interfere with social and professional functioning.

H_2-histamine receptor blockers have been tried with some success in patients who are not controlled on maximum doses of H_1-receptor blockers.

Tricyclic antidepressants with combined H_1- and H_2-blocking action, such as **doxepin** (Adapin, Sinequan) (maximum 300 mg/day), can be very effective, secondary to their combined antihistamine and antidepressant effect.

TOPICAL TACROLIMUS. Topical tacrolimus (Protopic) (previously known as FK506) is an immunosuppressant previously used systemically to control kidney graft rejection. Controlled studies have confirmed that topical tacrolimus (0.03% and 0.1% ointment, bid) is well tolerated and effective in the treatment of resistant AD in both adults and children. Marked improvement can frequently be observed within a week of initiating therapy, but many weeks of treatment are required for a sustained remission. Long-term side effects have not been evaluated yet, but systemic absorption of topical tacrolimus is associated with blood levels significantly lower than those associated with systemic administration. Recently, another topical immunosupressant (pimecrolimus topical 1%, Elidel) has also been approved for the treatement of AD in both adults and children. Topical tacrolimus and pimcrolimus are both increasingly becoming the preferred drugs for the initial treatment of moderate and severe AD.

ANTIBIOTIC AND OTHER ANTIMICROBIAL AGENTS. Antibiotic and other antimicrobial agents are definitely indicated in the presence of evident infection.

For localized impetigo-like lesions, topical mupirocin (Bactroban) can be used. Systemic cephalexin (Biocef, Keflex, Keftab, Zartan) or dicloxacillin (Dycill, Dynapen) are indicated if the infection is extensive. Some studies have shown benefit from **systemic antistaphylococcal therapy** (for 3–4 wks) in patients with resistant AD even in the absence of evidence of active infection.

Antifungal therapy (e.g., ketoconazole [Nizoral]) should be considered in adult patients with head, neck, and upper body resistant AD.

Vesicular lesions associated with flares may represent herpes simplex infection (**eczema herpeticum**). Small herpetic lesions usually resolve spontaneously, but larger or progressive lesions need PO or IV acyclovir (Zovirax).

ALTERNATIVE THERAPIES. Before the introduction of topical tacrolimus, oral cyclosporine (Neoral, Sandimmune), methotrexate (Rheumatrex, Trexall), azathioprine (Imuran), and phototherapy (psoralen/ultraviolet A; or combined ultraviolet A/ultraviolet B) have been used in cases of recalcitrant and steroid-resistant AD. These therapies have significant side-effect profiles. The indications for their use are much less compelling now that the efficacy and favorable side-effect profiles of topical tacrolimus and pimecrolimus have been established.

Hospitalization

Hospitalization may rarely be indicated in the treatment of AD. It can, however, be a useful adjunct to standard treatment under certain social conditions and in the presence of significant psychosocial dysfunction in the patient or his or her care providers. Hospitalization is also a very effective way of achieving environmental and dietary control. It frequently results in significant improvement in skin condition to allow for skin testing and DBPCFC.

Dietary Restriction

Dietary restriction should be considered in children with positive skin tests and/or RAST. DBPCFC is usually needed before implementation of strict elimination diets. Diet design should be evaluated carefully in consultation with a dietitian. Supplementation of vitamins, minerals, and essential nutrients in alternative forms is required to avoid malnutrition. In children, a 2-yr elimination period is required before reintroduction of restricted foods (one new food every 1–2 wks). Allergy to certain foods, such as peanuts and tree nuts, is a life-long and life-threatening condition, and these foods should not be reintroduced (see Chap. 16, Food Allergy and Other Adverse Food Reactions).

Immunotherapy

Immunotherapy was not found to be useful in AD and may even aggravate the skin condition. In adult patients, when immunotherapy is indicated for allergic rhinitis and bronchial asthma, it should be initiated at much lower extract concentrations than usual, with close observation of the skin condition.

Special Topics

Complications of Atopic Dermatitis

- Psychosocial: sleep disturbance, depression, anxiety, and behavioral problems.
- Eye complications: keratoconus, atopic keratoconjunctivitis, and anterior subcapsular cataract.
- Recurrent skin infections: staphylococcal, fungal, and eczema herpeticum.

Referral

Referral to a specialist is indicated in cases of uncertain diagnosis, severe or aggressive disease, oral steroid dependence, or complicated AD. The need for intensive patient education, allergy evaluations, and/or management of associated atopic disease are also indications for referral to an allergist.

KEY POINTS

- AD has a characteristic skin distribution that depends on the patient's age.
- Food allergies, especially egg and milk, contribute significantly to AD in approximately one-third of pediatric patients, but rarely in adult patients.
- Breaking the scratch-itch cycle is of utmost importance in the management of AD.
- Proper skin hydration and antihistamines are central to breaking the scratch-itch cycle.
- Topical tacrolimus or pimecrolimus are the preferred initial topical intervention in moderate and severe AD.
- Never use high-potency topical steroids on the face, genitals, or intertriginous skin.
- Oral corticosteroids should have no role in long-term management of AD.

SUGGESTED READING AND RESOURCES

Fleischer AB Jr. Treatment of atopic dermatitis: role of tacrolimus ointment as a topical noncorticosteroid therapy. *J Allergy Clin Immunol* 1999;104:S126–S130.

Grammer, LC. Atopic Dermatitis. In: Patterson R, Grammer LC, Greenberger PA, eds. *Allergic diseases diagnosis and management*, 5th ed. Lippincott Williams & Wilkins, 1997;305–310.

Hanifin JM, Tofte SJ. Update on therapy of atopic dermatitis. *J Allergy Clin Immunol* 1999;104:S123–S125.

Jaffe R. Atopic dermatitis. *Prim Care* 2000;27:503–513.

Jones SM, Burks AW Jr. Atopic Dermatitis. In: Lieberman P, Anderson J, eds. *Current clinical practice: allergic diseases: diagnosis and treatment*, 1st ed. Totowa, NJ: Humana Press, 1997;205–232.

Leung DYM, Diaz LA, DeLeo V, Soter NA. Allergic and immunologic skin disorders. In: Baker J, ed. *JAMA Primer on allergic and immunologic diseases*, 4th ed. Chicago: American Medical Association, 1997;1914–1923.

National Eczema Association for Science and Education, 1220 SW Morrison, Suite 433, Portland, OR 97205; Phone: 503-228-4430 or 800-818-7546; Internet address: http://eczema-assn.org.

REFERENCES

1. Hauk PJ, Hamid QA, Chrousos GP, Leung DY. Induction of corticosteroid insensitivity in human PBMCs by microbial superantigens. *J Allergy Clin Immunol* 2000;105(4):782–787.
2. Beltrani VS. The clinical spectrum of atopic dermatitis. *J Allergy Clin Immunol* 1999;104:S87–S98.

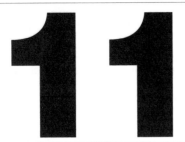

Allergic Contact Dermatitis

Barbara C. Jost

INTRODUCTION

Contact dermatitis is an eczematous dermatitis caused by exposure to an external agent.

Classification

Irritant Contact Dermatitis
Irritant contact dermatitis comprises 75% of all cases of contact dermatitis and is caused by direct tissue injury. It is not immunologically mediated. Common irritants include strong acids, alkalis, detergents, and organic solvents.

Allergic Contact Dermatitis
Allergic contact dermatitis (ACD) is immunologically mediated and requires prior sensitization. Approximately 25% of all contact dermatitis is of the allergic subtype. This chapter focuses primarily on ACD.

Epidemiology

Contact dermatitis and other eczemas were diagnosed during the course of over 7.1 million office visits and 430,000 hospital outpatient and emergency department encounters in 1996 [1]. It is estimated that ACD accounts for 7% of all occupation-related illnesses [2].

CAUSES

The **most common causes of ACD** in the United States are members of the *Rhus* genus (poison ivy, poison oak, poison sumac), paraphenylenediamine, nickel, rubber compounds, and ethylenediamine hydrochloride.

Pathophysiology

ACD is the result of a type IV, or **delayed-type hypersensitivity (DTH), reaction** (see Chap. 2, Basic Immunology Underlying Allergic Reactions and Allergic Inflammation). Recall that DTH reactions are mediated by T lymphocytes and not antibody. The first phase in the pathogenesis of ACD is *sensitization*. Subsequent exposures to the antigen trigger a series of events referred to as the *elicitation phase*.

Sensitization
Sensitization begins with topical application of the antigen. The antigen must penetrate the stratum corneum, where it is bound by Langerhans' cells or similar dendritic cells [antigen presenting cells (APCs)]. In the majority of instances, the APC migrates to draining lymph nodes via dermal lymphatics and presents antigen to helper T cells. Rarely, the APC–T cell interaction occurs in the skin. On presentation of antigen to helper T cells, clonal expansion and differentiation occur, resulting in the production of antigen-specific memory T cells that circulate systemically. The process

of sensitization takes approximately 4 days to complete. An individual may remain sensitized for many years.

Elicitation

On subsequent re-exposure, antigen is presented locally to sensitized CD4 helper T cells, which results in the release of proinflammatory cytokines [interleukin-1 (IL-1), IL-2, and interferon-gamma (IFN-gamma)] and chemokines within the skin. Macrophages, basophils, mast cells, and eosinophils are attracted to the site of challenge. It is important to note that DTH is a Th1 response (see Chap. 2, Basic Immunology of Allergic Reactions and Allergic Inflammation) and not a Th2 response. Hence, the relative contribution of basophils, mast cells, and eosinophils is minimal compared to lymphocytes, macrophages, and their respective cytokines.

Differential Diagnosis

Conditions that mimic ACD include irritant contact dermatitis, seborrheic dermatitis, nummular eczema, dyshidrotic eczema, and atopic dermatitis (see Chap. 10, Atopic Dermatitis). Patch testing (see Workup) may be the only means of distinguishing between ACD and irritant contact dermatitis.

PRESENTATION

History

Pruritus is a universal feature of ACD. The patient usually reports development of an erythematous rash followed by papules, and then pustules or vesicles. The interval between exposure to the causative agent and development of symptoms is 4–72 hrs, with most cases becoming symptomatic in 12–48 hrs.

It is important to take a careful social, occupational, and medical history to look for possible exposures to common sensitizing agents such as nickel, rubber (in particular, latex products), neomycin, poison ivy, and topical anesthetics.

Physical Exam

ACD can affect any area of the body. The scalp, palms, and soles are most resistant to contact sensitization, whereas areas subjected to friction, pressure, heat, and perspiration are more readily sensitized. The eyelids, neck, and genitalia are commonly sensitized.

The **pathognomonic** presentation is a rash at the site of contact with the antigen. A linear pattern is virtually pathognomonic for poison ivy.

The **appearance of the rash** depends on its stage at time of presentation. **Erythema** develops first, followed by **papules** and then pustules or **vesicles** and, in severe disease, **bullae**. Edema may be present and is particularly striking in the eyelids and genitalia. Borders are generally sharply demarcated. Subacutely, vesicles begin to involute, followed by crusting and scaling. Chronically, there is fissuring, thickening, and lichenification.

The **distribution of the rash** is one of the most helpful aids in identifying the causative allergen. Sparing of areas covered by clothing suggests an airborne allergen (e.g., ragweed oil, smoke from burning poison ivy), whereas involvement limited to clothed areas incriminates textile-related allergens. Dermatitis of the wrist, ear lobes, or neck may signify contact sensitivity to the nickel in jewelry. Involvement of only the head and neck may suggest a reaction to a component of hair dye, relaxers, or other cosmetic substance. ACD caused by nail polish tends to be localized to the eyelids (spread from hands). Involvement of the trunk and soles of the feet may indicate sensitization to rubber found in undergarments and shoes, respectively.

Many **systemically administered medications** can cross-react with structurally similar topical antigens and induce **generalized ACD** in a patient sensitized to the topical agent. An example is aminophylline, a complex of ethylenediamine and theophylline, which may cause a generalized reaction in patients previously sensitized to topical ethylenediamine, a stabilizer in some topical medications.

MANAGEMENT

Workup

If the identity of the sensitizing agent is not apparent after a thorough history and physical, then patch testing may be useful. Patch testing may also be used to confirm that a patient is sensitized to a suspected allergen. **Patch testing** involves the application of a panel of antigens, in nonirritating concentrations, to the skin (see Chap. 8, *In Vivo* and *In Vitro* Diagnostic Tests for Allergy, for further details).

A positive patch test means that the patient has been sensitized to the allergen tested. Positive patch test results must be correlated with history and physical to determine whether findings are indeed relevant to a past or present episode of dermatitis.

Treatment

Localized Reactions

- **Moist compresses** minimize oozing and facilitate absorption of topical steroids.
- Drying **antipruritic** lotions (e.g., calamine lotion) are simple and effective. Oral antihistamines may be necessary. Topical antihistamines and topical anesthetics should be avoided because of their sensitizing ability.
- **Topical corticosteroid creams,** not ointments, should be used.

Widespread Reactions

- **Systemic corticosteroids,** given at a dose of 40–60 mg initially, should be tapered slowly over 14 days to avoid flare-ups.
- **Oral antihistamines** (as for localized reactions) may be needed during the first few days of a course of systemic corticosteroids, particularly for pruritus that interrupts sleep.

Recurrence

Prevention of recurrence is predicated on avoidance (when possible). Patients should be educated about all possible sources of the allergen and potential cross-reacting substances.

KEY POINTS

- Allergic contact dermatitis is mediated by T lymphocytes.
- Rash distribution is the most helpful aid in identifying the causative allergen.

SUGGESTED READING

Belsito DV. The diagnostic evaluation, treatment, and prevention of allergic contact dermatitis in the new millennium. *J Allergy Clin Immunol* 2000;105(3):409–420.

Marks JG, Belsito DV, DeLeo VA, et al. North American Contact Dermatitis Group patch test results for the detection of delayed-type hypersensitivity to topical allergens. *J Am Acad Dermatol* 1998;38:911–918.

Samuels LG. Cutaneous allergy: allergic contact dermatitis and atopic dermatitis. In: Korenblat PE, Wedner HJ, eds. *Allergy: theory and practice*, 2nd ed. Philadelphia: WB Saunders, 1992;201–216.

REFERENCES

1. Centers for Disease Control and Prevention. Ambulatory care visits to physician offices, hospital outpatient departments and emergency departments: United States, 1996. National Center for Health Statistics Vital and Health Statistics Series, 1996;13(134).
2. Association of Schools of Public Health and National Institutes for Occupational Safety and Health. *Proposed national strategy for the prevention of leading work-related diseases and injuries, 2.* Washington, DC: The Association, 1988;65–95.

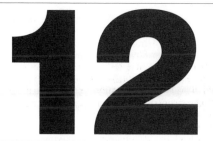

Ocular Allergic Diseases

Gregg J. Berdy and
Susan S. Berdy

INTRODUCTION

Ocular allergic diseases can be considered a spectrum of diseases ranging from mild itching and redness associated with seasonal allergic conjunctivitis to severe blinding sequelae secondary to atopic keratoconjunctivitis (AKC). The allergic ocular disorders can be categorized as seasonal allergic conjunctivitis, vernal keratoconjunctivitis (VKC), AKC, and giant papillary conjunctivitis (GPC).

CAUSES

Pathophysiology

Seasonal allergic conjunctivitis is the prototype of the group of diseases that begin as an antigen–IgE antibody interaction on the surface of conjunctival mast cells. Exposure of appropriately sensitized IgE-coated mast cells to airborne allergen is the initiating stimulus. The allergen binds two separate IgE molecules, creating a dimer formation that initiates the chain of reactions in the mast cell plasma membrane. The binding of mast cell IgE molecules causes the release of preformed mediators, such as histamine, and newly formed mediators that occur after the metabolism of arachidonic acid.

The sentinel role of histamine in the acute allergic response has been well established in the literature. The conjunctival surface contains both H_1-receptors and H_2-receptors, with each receptor subserving different roles in the ocular response to histamine. Stimulation of the H_1-receptor leads to symptoms of ocular itching, whereas stimulation of H_2-receptors produces vasodilation of conjunctival vessels.

Metabolism of arachidonic acid produces prostaglandins via the cyclooxygenase pathway and leukotrienes via the lipoxygenase pathway. Both prostaglandins and leukotrienes have been implicated in the promulgation of the ocular allergic response. Additionally, other mediators have been reported to participate in the ocular allergic process. Eosinophils release major basic protein, which has been shown to cause epithelial toxicity, and lymphocytes release interleukins, which have been demonstrated to promulgate the allergic response. T lymphocyte abnormalities have been demonstrated in AKC (Th1) and VKC (Th2).

Differential Diagnosis

The differential diagnosis of ocular allergic disorders includes any disease in which the eye becomes red with the associated symptoms of itching, burning, and tearing. There are both infectious and noninfectious etiologies. Therefore, the examining physician should be an astute observer when examining the ocular and periocular structures.

Infectious etiologies include viral, bacterial, and chlamydial entities. Viral infections are usually characterized by a unilateral red eye associated with a preauricular lymph node. Patients complain of matting of the eyelids with a clear to mucopurulent discharge. The conjunctiva displays follicular changes on the inferior tarsal surface. Often, the infection spreads to the opposite eye 3–9 days later. Patients may also have a concurrent upper respiratory infection.

Bacterial conjunctivitis is a disease that may present as a unilateral or bilateral condition in which patients develop eyelid erythema associated with conjunctival redness and chemosis. Patients usually complain of matting of the eyelids and a yellow to green purulent discharge. Exam of the ocular surface reveals a papillary reaction on the tarsal conjunctival surfaces and punctate keratopathy.

Whereas bacterial and viral conjunctivitis present with an acute onset, chlamydial infections are usually indolent and have been present for at least 6 wks before diagnosis. The patients present with a history of unilateral or bilateral conjunctival redness, associated with a foreign body sensation. Patients may have a follicular reaction in the lower lid but frequently are seen with a follicular/papillary reaction on the upper lids. Exam of the cornea may demonstrate superior or inferior pannus formation.

Noninfectious etiologies include contact dermatitis, drug-induced allergic contact dermatitis, keratoconjunctivitis sicca, and blepharitis. Contact dermatitis/conjunctivitis is usually caused by agents containing soaps, detergents, creams, lotions, cosmetics, or eye drops. Patients present with a contact dermatitis of the eyelids, as well as ocular irritation, redness, and itching. Exam of the inferior tarsal surface usually reveals a mixed papillary/follicular reaction.

Quite frequently, patients complaining of itching, burning, and red eyes have been diagnosed with "infections or allergies of the eyes," when in fact they may have external ocular diseases such as dry eye or blepharitis. The etiology of dry eye syndrome is myriad, as the tear film has three components: aqueous, lipid, and mucus. Any disease, such as blepharitis, meibomian gland dysfunction, keratoconjunctivitis sicca, or goblet cell dysfunction, that affects any of the tear film may lead to a functional dry eye.

MANAGEMENT

General Treatment

- Identify and remove offending allergen: pollen, mites, pets.
- Prevent circulating allergens from interacting with conjunctival mast cells, either by diluting the antigen load with tear substitutes or with immunotherapy.
- Suppress cellular and extracellular inflammation with the concomitant redness (vascular dilatation) and chemosis (edema) using vasoconstrictor agents, NSAIDs, and steroidal agents.
- Decrease itching and associated redness by using H_1-receptor antihistamines or antihistamine-vasoconstrictor combinations.
- Stabilize mast cell membranes to suppress or decrease inflammatory mediator release using oral and topical antihistamine and mast cell–stabilizing agents.

Allergic Conjunctivitis

- Avoidance, environmental control
- Irrigation with artificial tears
- Cool compresses
- Topical antihistamine/mast cell stabilizers
- Topical antihistamine/decongestants
- Topical selective H_1-receptor antagonists
- Topical mast cell stabilizers
- Topical steroids
- Rarely, systemic corticosteroids
- Occasionally, systemic antihistamines
- ?Allergen specific immunotherapy

Vernal Conjunctivitis

- Topical mast cell stabilizers
- Topical antihistamine/mast cell stabilizers
- Topical antihistamines

- Topical steroids
- Systemic antihistamines
- Occasionally requires short pulses of systemic steroids

Giant Papillary Conjunctivitis

- Discontinue lens wear for 3–6 wks
- Topical antihistamine/mast cell stabilizers
- Topical mast cell stabilizers during this time
- Topical steroids during this time
- Improve lens hygiene and fit
- Re-evaluate need for change in type of lens

Contact Dermatitis

- Avoidance of the allergen
- Topical antihistamines if conjunctival involvement
- Topical steroid (1% hydrocortisone cream) to eyelids
- Systemic antihistamines

Keratoconjunctivitis Sicca

- Tear replacement; consider preservative free
- Cautious use of oral antihistamines due to ocular drying from anticholinergic effects
- Slit lamp exam to evaluate meibomian glands/blepharitis lid scrubs and/or 6–12 mos of tetracycline or doxycycline
- Silicone punctual plugs

Disease Entities

Acute Allergic Conjunctivitis

Symptoms are bilateral, red, itching eyes associated with tearing and burning. Occasionally, a unilateral response may occur when there has been hand-to-eye contact with an allergen such as cat dander.

Physical exam reveals edematous and erythematous periocular tissues. The conjunctiva has mild to moderate chemosis with ropey mucous discharge in the tear film. The cornea is rarely involved. Approximately 70% of patients have an associated atopic disease such as allergic rhinitis, asthma, or atopic dermatitis.

Treatment of acute allergic conjunctivitis consists of

- Tear substitutes and cold compresses.
- Over-the-counter vasoconstrictor-antihistamine combinations such as Akon-A, Naphcon-A, Opcon-A, and Vasocon-A.
- Selective H_1-receptor antihistamines such as levocabastine (Livostin), emedastine (Emedine), and azelastine (Optivar).
- Combination H_1-receptor antihistamine/mast cell stabilizers such as olopatadine (Patanol) and ketotifen (Zaditor). These agents have been shown to be helpful in relieving the itching associated with allergic conjunctivitis, as well as having the additional benefit of suppressing ocular inflammation.
- NSAIDs, such as ketorolac (Acular), have been demonstrated to reduce ocular itching.
- Mast cell–stabilizing drugs can be used to inhibit the symptoms of allergic conjunctivitis and include cromolyn (Crolom), lodoxamide (Alomide), nedocromil (Alocril), and pemirolast (Alamast).
- Finally, topical steroid drops, such as loteprednol (Alrex), can be used for a short time with the caution of watching for increased intraocular pressure, corneal ulcers, and cataracts.

Vernal Conjunctivitis

Vernal conjunctivitis is usually seen in children ages 4–18, with a predilection for boys. Affected individuals frequently live in warm to hot, windy climates and have a strong family history of atopic disease. Patients may have perennial symptoms but usually have exacerbations during the spring and fall allergy seasons. Two subtypes of VKC exist—palpebral and limbal—and may occur singularly or simultaneously.

SYMPTOMS. Typically, a young boy presents with marked itching associated with a stringy, ropey mucus discharge. In severe cases, patients may complain of severe photophobia, pain, and, unfortunately, decreased visual acuity.

Physical exam reveals edematous and ptotic upper eyelids as a result of the marked inflammatory response. In patients with palpebral VKC, the upper tarsal surface develops large raised cobblestone papillae that are pathognomonic of the disease. These hypertrophic tissues are injected and may have mucus strands running in the crevices between them. In patients with limbal VKC, lid eversion reveals gelatinous elevations with whitish inclusions located at the limbus. These have been labeled *Horner-Trantas dots* and are an aggregation of eosinophils. Exam of the cornea in both forms of the disease may reveal superficial infiltrates and, in severe cases, epithelial defects with plaquelike deposition of material at the base. The lesions have been termed *shield ulcers*, which are usually located centrally just above the visual axis.

TREATMENT. As the potential for serious ocular sequelae exists with VKC, it is frequently necessary and appropriate to use a multifaceted treatment plan for controlling the disease. Controlling the itching is extremely important; children particularly tend to rub their eyes vigorously, which can induce mast cell degranulation and promulgate the disease process.

1. Identify and remove the offending allergen.
2. Topical antihistamines such as levocabastine, emedastine, or azelastine.
3. Topical antihistamine/mast cell stabilizers such as olopatadine or ketotifen.
4. NSAIDs, such as ketorolac, help relieve itching.
5. Mast cell stabilizers, such as cromolyn, lodoxamide, nedocromil, and pemirolast, have been useful as adjunctive therapy. These agents have been shown to improve the symptoms and associated corneal findings in patients treated for several weeks. Additionally, these drugs have been able to eliminate the need for or decrease the dependency on topical corticosteroid drops.
6. Pulsed therapy with topical corticosteroids, such as loteprednol (Alrex; Lotemax) or rimexolone (Vexol), is sometimes necessary to control inflammation.
7. Cool compresses, oral NSAIDs, and ASA have been shown to relieve the symptoms and signs of VKC.

Atopic Keratoconjunctivitis

AKC is a chronic disease usually seen in individuals in their fifth to sixth decade of life who have a long history of eczema or atopic dermatitis.

SYMPTOMS. Patients complain of chronic, year-round itching associated with burning, light sensitivity, tearing, and chronic redness of the eyes. The symptoms may go undiagnosed for years.

PHYSICAL EXAM. Exams of the patients show eczematoid changes of the upper and lower eyelids typified by induration, erythema, and scaling. Slit lamp exam reveals marked plugging of the meibomian gland orifices with purulent secretions and a concurrent poor precorneal tear film. The bulbar conjunctiva may show mild to moderate injection and changes consistent with keratoconjunctivitis sicca (dry eye). In severe cases, conjunctival subepithelial fibrosis and symblepharon may develop. The tarsal conjunctival surfaces usually reveal mild to moderate injection. Corneal involvement in AKC may vary according to the severity of disease. In mild forms, the cornea may only show minimal punctate stain with fluorescein dye, whereas severe cases demonstrate marked surface irregularity with epithelial desiccation associated with corneal neovascularization, keratinization, and scarring.

TREATMENT. Treatment must control both the skin and ocular surface inflammation and protect the corneal surface from the side effects of a poor tear film.

• To help open the plugged meibomian glands associated with severe blepharitis, hot compresses and oral antibiotics such as doxycycline, 100 mg bid, are used to help improve the meibomian gland dysfunction and subsequently improve the tear film. Antibiotics should have good coverage against staphylococcus bacteria.

- Preservative-free ocular lubricant drops or ointments help improve the aqueous deficiency of keratoconjunctivitis sicca.
- The lid scale component of blepharitis may be addressed with a combination of lid scrubs, using an over-the-counter preparation such as Eye-scrub or baby shampoo with water.
- For severe eczematoid changes, patients may benefit from topical 1% hydrocortisone cream or 0.03% tacrolimus ointment (Protopic) applied to the skin of the eyelids after using a nondrying soap such as Dove. Unscented lubricant creams, such as Eucerin, may be applied after the hydrocortisone cream to help hydrate the skin.
- Oral nonsedating antihistamines, such as Claritin, Allegra, and Zyrtec, are important to decrease the systemic allergic response.
- Topical H_1-receptor antagonist/mast cell stabilizers have been helpful in decreasing redness and inhibiting the itching associated with the disease.
- Mast cell–stabilizing agents may help.
- In severe cases where the corneal epithelial integrity has been violated, patients may need topical antibiotic eye drops to avoid infectious keratitis.
- Topical steroid drops may be used in patients who have severe corneal inflammation with vascularization.

Giant Papillary Conjunctivitis

GPC is a chronic inflammatory disorder related to exogenous materials causing chronic inflammation of the upper tarsal conjunctival surface. GPC has been noted in patients with ocular prostheses, patients with exposed nylon sutures, and, in most cases, secondary to contact lens wear. The etiology of this condition may be twofold: (a) poor lens edge design leading to chronic trauma to the upper tarsal conjunctiva and (b) antibody deposition on the contact lens surface leading to an antigen-antibody deposition on the contact lens surface leading to an antigen-antibody reaction in the upper tarsal conjunctiva.

SYMPTOMS. Patients present with complaints of chronic irritation, redness, and itching associated with decreased wearing time of their contact lenses. Eventually, patients may note increasing mucus discharge associated with pain, tearing, and hyperemia.

PHYSICAL EXAM. Exam may reveal minimal pathology, but over time, with chronic trauma to the upper tarsal conjunctival surfaces, hyperemia and giant papillae develop. The papillae are the result of chronic collagen deposition and tend to be more uniformly distributed, smaller, and flatter than those seen in the cobblestone appearance of patients with VKC. As the disease progresses, the cornea may show diffuse punctate keratitis or even corneal epithelial defects.

TREATMENT

1. Discontinue the offending agent—usually the contact lens. Initial therapy is to discontinue the patient's contact lenses for a brief period of time (1–3 wks).
2. Mast cell–stabilizing drugs and NSAIDs may be used in combination.
3. In patients with severe upper tarsal pathology, a topical corticosteroid eye drop may be necessary.
4. When contact lens wear is reintroduced, it is appropriate to use a lens with a better edge design or possibly change the composition of the lens material.

KEY POINTS

- The most important aspects of treating ocular allergic disease are a careful history taking and making a differential diagnosis.
- Rule out other causes of red, itchy eyes.
- Treat topical eye diseases topically.

SUGGESTED READING

Abelson MB, Allansmith MR. Histamine and the eye. In: Silverstein AM, O'Connor GR, eds. *Immunology and immunopathology of the eye. Proceeding of the second international symposium*, San Francisco, 1978. New York: Masson, 1979;362–364.

Abelson MB, Baird RS, Allansmith MR. Tear histamine levels in vernal conjunctivitis and other ocular inflammations. *Ophthalmology* 1980;87:812.

Abelson MB, Soter NA, Simon MA, et al. Histamine in human tears. *Am J Ophthalmol* 1977;83:417.

Abelson MB, Udell IJ. H_2-receptors in the human ocular surface. *Arch Ophthalmol* 1981;99:302.

Allansmith MR, Abelson MB. Ocular allergies. In: Smolin G, Thoft RA, eds. *The cornea*. Boston: Little, Brown, 1983;231–243.

Allansmith MR, Greiner JV, Baird RS. Number of inflammatory cells in the normal conjunctiva. *Am J Ophthalmol* 1978;86:250.

Ash ASF, Schild HO. Receptors mediating some actions of histamine. *Br J Pharmacol Chemotherapy* 1966;27:427.

Berdy GJ. Atopic keratoconjunctivitis. *Acta Ophthalmol Scand* 1999;77(suppl 228):7–9.

Berdy GJ. Ocular allergic disease in the senior patient: diagnosis and management. *Allergy Asthma Proc* 2000;21(5):277–283.

Berdy GJ. The effects of systemic medication on ocular allergic disease. *Acta Ophthalmol Scand* 2000;78:26–31.

Berdy GJ, Abelson MB, George MA, et al. Allergic conjunctivitis: a survey of new antihistamines. *J Ocular Pharm* 1991;7(4):313–324.

Berdy GJ, Hedqvist B. Ocular allergic disorders and dry eye disease: associations, diagnostic dilemmas and management. *Acta Ophthalmol Scand* 2000;78:32–37.

Berdy GJ, Spangler DL, Bensch G, et al. A comparison of the relative efficacy and clinical performance of olopatadine hydrochloride 0.1% ophthalmic solution and ketotifen fumarate 0.025% ophthalmic solution in the conjunctival antigen challenge model. *Clin Ther* 2000;22(7):826–833.

Black JW, Duncan WAM, Durant GJ, et al. Definition and antagonism of histamine H_2-receptors. *Nature* 1972;236:385.

Bradding P, et al. Interleukin-4 is localized to and released by human mast cells. *J Exp Med* 1992;176:1381.

Chabay R, et al. Receptor cross-linking and histamine release in basophils. *J Biol Chem* 1980;255:4628.

Craig SS, Schechter NM, Schwartz LB. Ultrastructural analysis of maturing human T and TC mast cells identified by immunoelectron microscopy. *Lab Invest* 1988;58:682.

Denburg JA, Silver JE, Abrams JS. Interleukin-5 is a human basophilopoietin: induction of histamine content and basophilic differentiation of HL-60 cells and of peripheral blood basophil-eosinophil progenitors. *Blood* 1991;77:1462.

Dvorak AM, Galli SJ, Schulman ES, et al. Basophil and mast cell degranulation: ultrastructural analysis of mechanisms of mediator release. *Federation Proc* 1983; 42:2510.

Flowers RJ, Blackwell GJ. The importance of phospholipase A_2 in prostaglandin biosynthesis. *Biochem Pharmacol* 1976;25:285.

Foreman FC, Hallet MB, Mangar J. The relationship between histamine secretion and ^{45}calcium uptake by mast cells. *J Physiol* 1977;271:193.

Gell PGH, Coombs RRA. *Clinical aspects of immunology*, 2nd ed. Oxford: Blackwell Scientific Publishers, 1968;575–596.

Goetzl EJ, Weller PF, Valone FH. Biochemical and functional basis of the regulatory and protective roles of the human eosinophil. In: Weissmann G, Samuelsson B, Paoletti R, eds. *Advances in inflammation research*. New York: Raven, 1979;157.

Harvey RP, Schocket AL. The effect of H_1 and H_2 blockade on cutaneous histamine response in man. *J Allergy Clin Immunol* 1980;65:136.

Heavy DJ, et al. Generation of leukotriene C4, leukotriene B4, and prostaglandin D2 by immunologically activated rat intestinal mucosal mast cells. *J Immunol* 1988;140:1953.

Holgate ST, et al. Relationship between mediator release form human lung mast cells in vitro and in vivo. *Int Arch Allergy Appl Immunol* 1985;77:47.

Irani AA, Schwartz LB. Mast cell heterogeneity. *Clin Exp Allergy* 1989;19:143.

Ishizaka T, Ishizaka K. Biology of immunoglobulin E: molecular basis of reaginic hypersensitivity. *Prog Allergy* 1975;19–60.

Ishizaka T, Hirata F, Sterk AR, et al. Bridging of IgE receptors activates phospholipid methylation and adenylate cyclase in mast cell plasma membranes. *Proc Natl Acad Sci U S A* 1981;78:6812.

Ishizaka T, et al. Biochemical analysis of initial triggering events of IgE-mediated histamine release from human lung mast cells. *J Immunol* 1983;130:2357.

Lagunoff D. Membrane fusion during mast cell secretion. *J Cell Biol* 1973;57:252.

Levene RZ. Mast cells and amines in normal ocular tissues. *Invest Ophthalmol* 1962;1:531.

Lewis RA, Austen KF, Soberman RJ. Leukotrienes and other products of the 5-lipoxygenase pathway. *N Engl J Med* 1990;323:645.

Lewis RA, et al. Prostaglandin D2 generation after activation of rat and human mast cells with anti-IgE. *J Immunol* 1982;129:1627.

McNeil HP, Austen KF. Biology of the mast cell. In: Frank MM, Austen KF, Claman HN, Unanue ER, eds. *Samter's immunologic diseases*, 5th ed. Boston: Little, Brown, 1995;185–204.

Ravetch JV, Kinet J-P. Fc receptors. *Annu Rev Immunol* 1991;9:457.

Riley JF, West GB. The presence of histamine in tissue mast cells. *J Physiol (London)* 1953;120:528.

Schwartz LB. Monoclonal antibodies against human mast cell tryptase demonstrate shared antigenic sites on subunits of tryptase and selective localization of the enzyme to mast cells. *J Immunol* 1985;134:526.

Schwartz LB, Austen KF. Structure and function of the chemical mediators of mast cells. *Prog Allergy* 1984;34:271.

Siraganian RP, Hook WA, Levine BB. Specific *in vitro* histamine release from basophils by bivalent haptens: evidence for activation by simple bridging of membrane bound antibody. *Immunochemistry* 1975;12:149.

Smith JA, Mansfield LE, deShazo R, Nelson HS. An evaluation of the pharmacologic inhibition of the immediate and late cutaneous effects to allergen. *J Allergy Clin Immunol* 1980;65:118.

Smelser GK, Silver S. The distribution of mast cells in the normal eye. A method of study. *Exp Eye Res* 1963;2:134.

Sommerhoff CP, et al. Mast cell chymase: a potent secretagogue for airway gland serous cells. *J Immunol* 1989;142:2450.

Soter NA, et al. Local effects of synthetic leukotrienes (LTC4, LTD4, LTE4 and LTB4) in human skin. *J Invest Dermatol* 1983;80:115.

Weston JH, Udell IJ, Abelson MB. H_1 receptors in the human ocular surface. *Invest Ophthalmol Vis Sci* 1981;20(suppl):32.

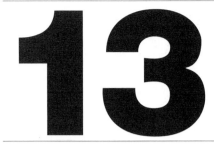

Anaphylaxis

Barbara C. Jost

INTRODUCTION

Anaphylaxis is a medical emergency. It refers to a constellation of systemic signs and symptoms that is the result of the IgE–dependent release of vasoactive mediators in response to an allergen. Anaphylaxis requires timely and decisive management. It is rapid in evolution and may be deadly.

There are an estimated 500 fatal anaphylactic reactions/yr in the United States.

The most common allergens provoking anaphylaxis are drugs, in particular beta-lactams; Hymenoptera stings; and foods (crustaceans and peanuts). Immunotherapy, latex, and, rarely, insect bites (other than Hymenoptera stings) are other known causes.

Anaphylactoid reactions are not IgE-dependent but are due to the direct release of mediators from mast cells. Clinical manifestations and management are the same as for anaphylactic reactions.

Radiocontrast medium is the most common cause of anaphylactoid reactions (Table 13-1).

CAUSES

Pathophysiology

Anaphylaxis is a **type I, or immediate hypersensitivity** (see Chap. 2, Basic Immunology Underlying Allergic Reactions and Allergic Inflammation) reaction. It is elicited by the cross-linking of allergen-specific IgE bound to the surface of mast cells and basophils by allergen.

Mediators
The cross-linking promotes the release of histamine, leukotrienes, enzymes, and other vasoactive mediators from mast cells and basophils. Histamine by itself causes vascular smooth muscle relaxation and increased microvascular permeability. The effects of histamine are potentiated by the leukotrienes.

Differential Diagnosis

When only a single sign or symptom occurs during a suspected episode of anaphylaxis, such as flushing, bronchospasm, or cramping, it is difficult to delineate a nonimmunologic or idiosyncratic reaction from true anaphylaxis. A number of conditions can mimic anaphylaxis. The vasovagal reaction is most often mistaken for anaphylaxis; other diagnoses to consider are outlined in Table 13-2.

PRESENTATION

Risk Factors

- History of anaphylaxis
- Parenteral exposure to antigen

TABLE 13-1. COMMON CAUSES OF ANAPHYLACTOID REACTIONS

Radiocontrast medium

ASA, NSAIDs

Opiates

IV immunoglobulin

Vancomycin (red man syndrome)

Scromboid fish poisoning

Blood products (e.g., in immunoglobulin A–deficient patients)

Exercise

Idiopathic

- Intermittent exposure to antigen
- Large dose exposure

Adults are at higher risk for anaphylaxis due to penicillin and Hymenoptera, whereas children are at higher risk for food-induced anaphylaxis.

Atopy does not appear to increase the risk of anaphylaxis, but it may place an individual at risk for more severe expressions of anaphylaxis, including death.

Beta-blocker therapy places the individual at risk for a more severe anaphylaxis reaction and may make resuscitation more difficult.

History and Physical Exam

Anaphylaxis is an acute, life-threatening syndrome involving multiple organ systems.

Onset of symptoms is typically within minutes of exposure to antigen, although in rare circumstances it can be delayed for hours. Median time to collapse is 30 mins for food exposure and 5 mins for a parenterally administered agent [1].

A delayed reaction can occur in some individuals (**biphasic reaction**), leading to recurrence of symptoms 4–8 hrs after the initial event.

Protracted anaphylaxis requiring many hours of active resuscitation occurs in as many as 28% of patients [2]. Risk factors for prolonged anaphylaxis are oral ingestion of the allergen and onset of symptoms more than 30 mins after exposure to the stimulus.

The presentation of anaphylaxis is highly variable. Signs and symptoms include any combination of the following: flushing, hypotension, loss of consciousness, bron-

TABLE 13-2. DIFFERENTIAL DIAGNOSIS OF ANAPHYLAXIS

Vasovagal reaction

Drug overdose

Adrenal insufficiency

Serotonin syndrome (e.g., carcinoid syndrome)

Panic attack

Sepsis syndrome

Cardiogenic shock

Arrhythmias

Hypoglycemia

Other causes of angioedema: ACE inhibitors, hereditary angioedema

chospasm, tachycardia, urticaria, angioedema, laryngeal edema, abdominal or uterine cramping, diarrhea, vomiting, pruritus, rhinorrhea/sneezing, conjunctival injection. Reactions can range from mild to severe.

Anaphylaxis can be a feature of **systemic mastocytosis** (see Chap. 19, Mastocytosis).

MANAGEMENT

Workup

Lab Testing

If the diagnosis of anaphylaxis is in question, it is possible to measure a serum **beta-tryptase level**. *Remember to stabilize the patient first and draw a beta-tryptase level later.* Studies have shown that increased levels of beta-tryptase correspond to acute mediator release. In the case of an insect sting anaphylaxis, beta-tryptase blood levels are maximal 15–120 mins after anaphylaxis and decline with a half-life of 1.5–2.5 hrs [3]. Practically speaking, beta-tryptase levels are measurable for up to 8 hrs (with newer assays) after a putative anaphylactic reaction.

Skin Testing

Patients are often referred to an allergist after an episode of presumed anaphylaxis. If a careful history uncovers the causative agent, then confirmatory skin testing, *in vitro* testing or challenge testing (see Chap. 8, *In Vivo* and *In Vitro* Diagnostic Tests for Allergy) can be offered to the patient. Limitations and risks of testing should be discussed with the patient. *Skin tests are not reliable for up to 4–6 wks after an episode of anaphylaxis.* A single episode of anaphylaxis with no obvious causative antigen by history does not warrant random skin testing or *in vitro* testing.

Recurrent Episodes

Recurrent episodes of anaphylaxis without a known antigen warrant consideration of other diagnoses. If no alternative diagnosis is identified, then **systemic mastocytosis** should be considered (see Chap. 19, Mastocytosis); total (alpha + beta) tryptase levels are persistently elevated in this condition even when the patient is asymptomatic. If features are not compatible with systemic mastocytosis, then a diagnosis of **idiopathic anaphylaxis** may be considered. Idiopathic anaphylaxis is a *diagnosis of exclusion* when no identifiable causative factors can be found for an episode of anaphylaxis. It is the result of nonimmunologic mast cell activation. The acute presentation and treatment are the same as for anaphylaxis due to known allergens. Patients who have more than 6 episodes/yr may be candidates for maintenance prednisone therapy.

Treatment

Regardless of severity, all anaphylactic reactions deserve treatment and observation, as any mild reaction can rapidly degrade into a more serious reaction.

Epinephrine

Epinephrine is the cornerstone of management (Fig. 13-1). It should be administered immediately using a dose of 0.3–0.5 mg IM (0.3–0.5 mL of a 1:1,000 solution) in the thigh (vastus medialis) or upper extremity (deltoid). Epinephrine may be repeated at 5-min intervals as necessary.

Smaller doses may be needed in the **elderly** (e.g., 0.2 mg).

Larger doses (0.5 mg) are typically needed in patients receiving **beta-blockers**. Glucagon (1–2 mg IV push) may be needed in these patients.

Administration via **central line** (3–5 mL of 1:10,000 solution) or through an **endotracheal tube** (3–5 mL of a 1:10,000 solution diluted in 10 mL normal saline) may be necessary in cases of severe hypotension or respiratory failure.

A **continuous infusion** of 1:10,000 epinephrine may be necessary in patients with protracted symptoms. Potential risks of IV epinephrine include myocardial ischemia

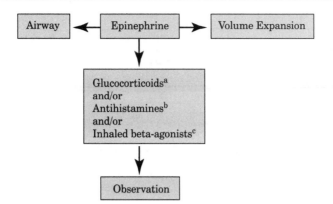

FIG. 13-1. Management of anaphylaxis. [a]methylprednisolone, 125 mg IV, or hydrocortisone, 500 mg IV. [b]H_1 and H_2 antagonists in combination: diphenhydramine, 50 mg IM or IV, + cimetidine, 300 mg IV. [c]albuterol, 0.5 mL in 2.5 mL normal saline, for resistant bronchospasm.

and infarction, arrhythmia, and hypertensive crisis. Keeping these risks in mind, a bolus of 100–200 μg/70 kg over a period of 5–10 mins may be given (1:10,000 concentration). A continuous infusion of 1–5 μg/minute/70 kg is usually sufficient to maintain BP.

A second injection (0.1–0.2 mg of a 1:1,000 solution) may be given **directly into the site** of an insect sting or drug injection to delay systemic absorption of the allergen, as long as the site is not a digit or other terminal part of the anatomy.

Airway Management
Airway management may require endotracheal intubation. Racemic epinephrine via metered dose inhaler may be useful in treating laryngeal edema. If laryngeal edema is severe and not immediately responsive to epinephrine, consider cricothyroidotomy or tracheotomy.

Volume Expansion
Volume expansion with IV fluids, beginning with a 500- to 1,000-mL bolus, should be titrated to BP and urine output. Colloid solutions, such as hetastarch (Hespan) and serum albumin, may be beneficial in cases of refractory hypotension or shock. The risk-benefit profile of each solution should be carefully weighed, as hetastarch may prolong bleeding times and albumin may precipitate pulmonary edema.

Glucocorticoids
Glucocorticoids do not have an immediate effect but may prevent relapse of symptoms.

Antihistamines
Antihistamines also will not have an immediate impact on the course of anaphylaxis, but they may shorten the duration of symptoms. Diphenhydramine (Benadryl) can be administered IV (25–100 mg over 5–10 mins), IM, or PO. It can be given every 6 hrs for 24–48 hrs after the reaction. H_2-antagonists (e.g., ranitidine, cimetidine) may also be added [4].

Observation
Patients with mild reactions limited to flushing, urticaria, angioedema, cramping, or mild bronchospasm should be monitored in the emergency department for a minimum of 6–8 hrs. All others warrant admission to hospital for 24-hr observation.

Follow-Up: Prevention

Secondary prevention is predicated on **identification and avoidance** of the offending antigen. Accidental ingestion of allergenic foods in the form of condiments and prepared foods is a well-known hazard, particularly for food-allergic children (see Chap. 16, Food Allergy and Other Adverse Food Reactions).

Patients with a history of anaphylaxis due to food or a Hymenoptera sting should carry **self-administered epinephrine** (e.g., Epi Pen or Ana-Kit).

Desensitization in the use case of certain drugs (see Chap. 14, Drug Allergy and Desensitization) or **immunotherapy** in the case of venom should be considered if future exposure to the putative agent is unavoidable.

- Immunotherapy with Hymenoptera venom is highly efficacious (85–98%) (see Chap. 15, Insect Allergy).
- Immunotherapy is not recommended for food-induced anaphylaxis.

KEY POINTS

- Anaphylaxis is an acute, life-threatening syndrome involving multiple organ systems.
- Drugs, foods, and Hymenoptera are the most common causes of anaphylaxis.
- Epinephrine is the cornerstone of management.

SUGGESTED READING AND RESOURCES

Corren J, Schocket AL. Anaphylaxis: a preventable emergency. *Postgrad Med* 1990; 7(5):167–168, 171–178.

The JCAAI website at http://www.jcaai.org/Param/Anaphylax.htm for practice parameters for anaphylaxis.

Kemp SF, Lockey RF, Wolf BL, Lieberman P. Anaphylaxis. A review of 266 cases. *Arch Intern Med* 1995;155(16):1749–1754.

Ring J, Behrendt H. Anaphylaxis and anaphylactoid reactions. Classification and pathophysiology, 1999. *Clin Rev Allergy Immunol* 17(4):387–389.

Sim TC. Anaphylaxis: how to manage and prevent this medical emergency. *Postgrad Med* 1992;92(5):277–284, 289, 292–296 [erratum appears in *Postgrad Med* 1993;93 (1):16].

Wyatt R. Anaphylaxis: how to recognize, treat, and prevent potentially fatal attacks. *Postgrad Med* 1996;100(2):87–90, 96–99.

REFERENCES

1. Pumphrey RS. Lessons for management of anaphylaxis from a study of fatal reactions. *Clin Exp Allergy* 2000;30(8):1144–1150.
2. Stark BJ, Sullivan TJ. Biphasic and protracted anaphylaxis. *J Allergy Clin Immunol* 1985;78:76–83.
3. Schwartz LB, Irani AA. Serum tryptase and the laboratory diagnosis of mastocytosis. *Hematol Oncol Clin North Am* 2000;14(3):641–657.
4. Ring J, Behrendt H. H1- and H2-antagonists in allergic and pseudoallergic diseases. *Clin Exp Allergy* 1990;20(Suppl 2):43–49.

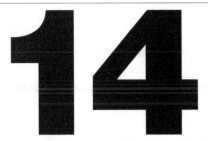

Drug Allergy and Desensitization

Barbara C. Jost

INTRODUCTION

Drug allergy or hypersensitivity is a form of **adverse drug reaction** (ADR).

Definition

An *ADR* is defined as any undesirable effect of a drug beyond its intended or beneficial effects. Most ADRs are predictable and may occur in any normal individual exposed to a drug, if a sufficient dose is given. The spectrum is broad and includes side effects, drug interactions, and overdose. Those ADRs that are not predictable and occur in a smaller subset of the general population include drug intolerance, idiosyncrasy, and immunologic drug reactions, or **drug allergies**.

Epidemiology

It is estimated that up to 15% of drug administrations culminate in an ADR; the risk is roughly doubled in the hospital setting [1]. Fatal drug reactions occur in approximately 0.1% of medical inpatients [2] and 0.01% of surgical inpatients [3]. Immunologic drug reactions, or allergic drug reactions, as we refer to them in this text, account for only 5–10% of all ADRs [4].

Approach to the Patient with Allergic Drug Reaction

The approach to a patient presenting with a possible allergic drug reaction begins with thorough history taking and information gathering:

1. What were the signs and symptoms? In what order did they appear and resolve? Pay particular attention to manifestations compatible with an immunologic etiology such as urticaria and angioedema.
2. What was the time course of the putative reaction? For example, onset relative to first dose of drug, time to peak reaction, time to resolution after discontinuing therapy.
3. Why was the drug prescribed? Can any signs or symptoms be explained by intercurrent illness, e.g., viral exanthems are often mistaken for allergic drug reactions.
4. What other drugs was the patient taking at the time of the putative reaction? It is important to consider all drugs taken by the patient at the time of the reaction as possible offenders, regardless of the duration of administration or a history of apparent tolerance to the drug. Remember to also ask about over-the-counter drugs and dietary supplements.
5. Has the patient ever received the drug, or drugs in the same or a related class, before? If so, how long ago, and what was the outcome?
6. Survey the patient's medication list for drugs with established allergic potential. Search pharmocologic reference books (e.g., *Physicians' Desk Reference* [5]) and the medical literature for information on the incidence and expression of allergic reactions involving other drugs on the patient's list.
7. Does the patient report a history of other allergic drug reactions?

Many allergy consults arise when a patient with a history of a specific drug allergy requires treatment with that drug or a closely related drug, e.g., a patient with history of penicillin allergy develops a multiple drug-resistant infection susceptible only to a beta-lactam antibiotic. In cases such as these, the following information in also important:

1. When did the reaction occur? Hypersensitivity wanes with time. Only 40% of patients with a history of penicillin allergy and a positive skin test will continue to have a positive skin test 5 yrs later [6].
2. Has the patient taken the drug in question, a drug in the same class, or a drug with a similar chemical structure since then? What was the outcome in each instance?
3. Has the patient undergone prior evaluation by an allergist? In the case of a beta-lactam antibiotic, was the patient skin tested?

CAUSES

Pathophysiology
Allergic drug reactions are usually defined as reactions caused by proved or suspected immunologic mechanisms. Allergic drug reactions result from the production of antibodies and/or cytotoxic T cells directed against the drug, its metabolite, or the combination of the drug and a soluble or cell-bound carrier protein. These immunologic responses are produced in response to prior or continuous exposure to a drug or an antigenically related agent.

Complete Antigens
High-molecular-weight (HMW) drugs like insulin can induce the production of antidrug antibodies without the need to couple to a carrier protein, thus acting as "complete antigens." HMW drugs are more likely to provoke an allergic reaction than low-molecular-weight (LMW) drugs.

Haptens
Most drugs are LMW agents and cannot induce an immune response; they are not complete antigens. These drugs or their biotransformed metabolites (e.g., penicillin metabolites) act as haptens and must first covalently combine with carrier proteins in the body to elicit an immune response. The actual allergen may be the hapten itself, the hapten-protein complex, or a tissue protein that has been altered by interaction with the drug and is then recognized as foreign.

Immunologic Mechanisms
The immunologic mechanisms of drug allergy can be stratified according to the Gell and Coombs classification of hypersensitivity (see Chap. 2, Basic Immunology Underlying Allergic Reactions and Allergic Inflammation). Numerous other reactions are thought to have an immunologic basis, although the exact mechanism is unknown. Still others behave like immunologic reactions but are not.

- **Type I** (IgE-mediated or immediate hypersensitivity—e.g., anaphylaxis): The time course is usually seconds to minutes for drugs administered parenterally and up to 1 hr for drugs taken orally.
- **Type II** (antibody-dependent cytotoxic hypersensitivity) is typified by hemolytic anemia due to antibodies formed against cell-bound drugs, such as erythrocyte-bound penicillin.
- **Type III** (immune-complex-mediated hypersensitivity) is typified by serum sickness syndrome.
- **Type IV** (delayed-type, hypersensitivity, T cell mediated) may manifest as a granulomatous reaction or contact dermatitis.
- Mechanism unknown (presumed immunologic): Examples include Stevens-Johnson syndrome, toxic epidermal necrolysis, drug fever, acute interstitial nephritis, and pulmonary infiltrates with eosinophilia.

TABLE 14-1. HOST FACTORS INFLUENCING DRUG IMMUNOGENICITY

Positive influence	No influence
Age (adults > children and very old)	Family history of atopy
Gender (females > males)	Atopy (beta-lactams)
Presence of infection	
History of reaction to any drug	
Personal or family history of multiple drug allergies	
Atopy (in the case of NSAIDs)	

- **Anaphylactoid** or "pseudoallergic" reactions are clinically indistinguishable from anaphylactic reactions but are not IgE-mediated (see Chap. 13, Anaphylaxis). Opiates and radiocontrast media are examples of agents that induce anaphylactoid reactions with release of histamine independent of IgE.

Factors influencing immunologic drug reactions include the following:

- Route of administration (parenteral more immunogenic than PO)
- Dosing (higher doses > lower doses)
- Time interval (shorter intervals > longer intervals)
- Timing of doses (multiple intermittent doses > single dose)
- Drug structure (HMW > LMW)
- Ability to bind self proteins (greater binding is more immunogenic)
- Numerous host characteristics (Table 14-1).

PRESENTATION

Physical Exam

Alterations in the skin and mucous membranes are the most common manifestation of drug hypersensitivity.

Maculopapular or Morbilliform Skin Eruptions
Maculopapular or morbilliform skin eruptions are seen most often. Drug classes associated with maculopapular rash include beta-lactam antibiotics, sulfonamides, anticonvulsants, and NSAIDs. The rash tends to be symmetric in distribution, sparing palms and soles. It is often confluent and consists of erythematous macules and papules. Onset is approximately 4–7 days into a course of therapy, beginning on the lower extremities or over pressure points. Maculopapular rash occurs in 2–3% of patients receiving penicillin. The frequency of rash approaches 10% with ampicillin; it is nearly universal when ampicillin is given in the setting of Epstein-Barr virus infection. For unknown reasons, this rash also occurs in 70% of patients with chronic lymphocytic leukemia given ampicillin and in a similar proportion among patients also taking allopurinol. In the case of ampicillin rash, skin tests are typically negative. The mechanism of maculopapular drug rash is disputed; two proposed mechanisms are IgM immune complex formation and cell-mediated (type IV) hypersensitivity [7].

Urticaria and Angioedema
Urticaria and angioedema (see Chap. 9, Urticaria and Angiodema) are classic examples of type I, or immediate hypersensitivity. Onset and resolution are typically quite rapid, although resolution can take weeks in some cases.

Fixed Drug Eruptions
Fixed drug eruptions are macular, nonpruritic, violaceous skin eruptions that occur at the same location on the body with each exposure to a given drug. Common offending

drugs include phenolphthalein, analgesics, barbiturates, beta-lactam antibiotics, sulfonamides, and tetracycline.

Contact Dermatitis
Contact dermatitis (see Chap. 11, Allergic Contact Dermatitis) occurs primarily in relation to cutaneous exposure and hence is seen only with topically applied drugs. Orally and parenterally administered agents can potentially cause a contact dermatitis in nurses, pharmacists, and persons involved in drug manufacture.

Interstitial Granulomatous Dermatitis
Interstitial granulomatous dermatitis is characterized by violaceous plaques with a predilection for skin folds. The mechanism is thought to be delayed-type hypersensitivity to drugs, such as ACE inhibitors and furosemide.

Erythema Multiforme
Erythema multiforme is a polymorphic skin eruption presenting with any combination of macules, papules, vesicles, bullae, and targetoid lesions. An estimated 10–20% of cases are related to drugs, including sulfonamides, penicillin, barbiturates, salicylates, and antimalarials.

Erythema Multiforme Major (Stevens-Johnson Syndrome)
A febrile form of erythema multiforme, termed *erythema multiforme major*, or *Stevens-Johnson syndrome*, is characterized by fever, **mucous membrane involvement**, and sloughing of up to 10% of the epidermis. Treatment involves removal of the offending agent and prompt use of systemic steroids. Corticosteroids have been shown to reduce morbidity and improve outcome for Stevens-Johnson syndrome [8]. Readministration of the presumed offending drug results in recurrence of the syndrome, hence *drug challenge (even graded challenge) is contraindicated*.

Toxic Epidermal Necrolysis
Toxic epidermal necrolysis (TEN) is a life-threatening febrile illness characterized by diffuse necrosis and sloughing of cutaneous and mucosal epithelial surfaces (>30% of the epidermal surface). Visceral involvement accounts for a mortality rate of up to 40% [9]. As with Stevens-Johnson syndrome, a *history of TEN precludes drug challenge* with the putative drug.

Serum Sickness Syndrome
Serum sickness syndrome is ascribed to soluble immune complexes (type III hypersensitivity). The syndrome encompasses a broad spectrum of signs and symptoms, including fever, malaise, rash (palpable purpura and urticaria), lymphadenopathy, leukopenia, arthralgias/myalgias, and arthritis. The syndrome begins within 2–4 wks of drug ingestion and resolves only when the offending agent or its metabolite is completely eliminated from the body.

Systemic Lupus Erythematosus–Like Drug Reactions
SLE–like drug reactions are due to circulating immune complexes. Drugs causing a lupus-like reaction include hydralazine, procainamide, isoniazid, and phenytoin.

Drug Fever
Drug fever may be the only evidence of hypersensitivity to a drug. It typically develops around day 7–10 and disappears within 36–72 hrs [10] after the drug is stopped, although it can persist for days. The fever often reaches high levels. Associated findings may include eosinophilia, leukocytosis, rash, and an elevated ESR. The mechanism is unknown.

Hematologic Manifestations
Hematologic manifestations of drug allergy (type II hypersensitivity) include the following:

- Coombs positive hemolytic anemia (penicillin, phenacetin, methyldopa, quinidine)

- Thrombocytopenia (quinine, quinidine, sulfonamides, heparin)
- Neutropenia (phenylbutazone, penicillin, antithyroid drugs)

Corticosteroids may decrease the severity of hematologic reactions in some cases.

Drug-Induced Hepatitis
Drug-induced hepatitis has been linked to over 150 different drugs. It begins after several weeks of drug treatment and recurs rapidly on rechallenge. Patterns of liver damage include hepatocellular and cholestatic; both types of damage can occur simultaneously. Clinical findings may include fever, rash, lymphadenopathy, hemolysis, and eosinophilia. Drug-induced hepatitis does not appear to be dose-dependent. Common causative agents include isoniazid, halothane, phenytoin, amoxicillin-clavulanate, and the sulfonamides [11].

Acute Interstitial Nephritis
Acute interstitial nephritis is rare but can be seen with beta-lactam antibiotics, in particular methicillin, as well as rifampin, NSAIDs, sulfonamides, captopril, and allopurinol. It is associated with fever, rash, and eosinophilia. Hematuria, albuminuria, pyuria, an active sediment, elevated serum creatinine, and even oliguria have been noted. Biopsy shows a mononuclear infiltrate with eosinophilia and tubular damage. Two investigators have demonstrated IgG in the interstitium [12,13].

Anaphylaxis
See Chap. 13, Anaphylaxis.
    Beta-lactam antibiotics are the most frequent known cause of anaphylaxis.

MANAGEMENT
Management of drug allergy is complicated by limited available diagnostic tests and the increased risks and costs associated with the use of alternative agents.

Diagnostic Testing

Skin Testing
See Chap. 8, *In Vivo* and *In Vitro* Diagnostic Tests for Allergy.
    The detection of drug-specific IgE antibody by *in vivo* testing (skin testing) [or *in vitro* testing (RAST or ELISA)] requires knowledge of the chemical structure of the immunogen, typically a metabolite of the suspect drug. This is known for only a handful of drugs; the best-studied and most reliable are penicillin and the first-generation cephalosporins. LMW drugs, such as toxoids, antisera, and egg-protein vaccines, are complete antigens and can be used directly as skin-testing reagents. However, protocols are not standardized, and positive responses must be distinguished from irritant (false-positive) responses. *Skin tests are not valid for 2–4 wks after an episode of acute anaphylaxis (refractory period).*

Patch Testing
Patch testing is used to assess for type IV contact hypersensitivity to topical agents. A panel of antigens is applied to the skin under an occlusive dressing, and the results are read at 48–72 hrs. See Chap. 8, *In Vivo* and *In Vitro* Diagnostic Tests for Allergy.

In Vitro *Studies*
In vitro studies are of varying degrees of usefulness in the assessment of drug allergy.

- **Beta-tryptase levels** remain elevated for up to 8 hrs after a putative anaphylactic event and are more sensitive than serum or urine histamine levels (see Chap. 13, Anaphylaxis).
- Decreases in total hemolytic complement (CH_{50}) or C3 and C4 levels may be seen in association with drug reactions causing complement activation.
- Total serum IgE levels are not useful for drug allergy.

- **RAST** measures drug-specific IgE antibody levels (see Chap. 8, *In Vivo* and *In Vitro* Diagnostic Tests for Allergy). It has been available for the major antigenic determinants of penicillin since 1971.
  - **Sensitivity:** RAST is less sensitive than skin testing for penicillin allergy, eliciting positive results in 60–95% of patients with a positive skin test to the major determinant of penicillin [14]. It is also more time consuming and requires specialized lab services. The RAST has been developed for numerous drugs, including insulin, muscle relaxants, thiopental, and trimethoprim, but sensitivity and specificity are variable. Caution must be exercised in ordering commercially available RASTs, as some labs offer testing for drugs that are not even associated with IgE-mediated allergic reactions.

- Direct drug challenge can be used to confirm that ingestion of a suspect drug causes a specific sign or symptom. This approach carries the risk of a potentially serious adverse reaction and is generally not recommended.

Treatment

- Discontinue (or substitute with a non–cross-reacting agent) all drugs that have both a temporal relationship to the putative allergic reaction and known allergic potential. Monitor the patient for resolution of signs and symptoms.
- Consider skin testing if available and reliable.
- Consider provocative dose challenge (under strict medical supervision) or desensitization (in the case of an IgE-mediated allergic reaction or positive skin test) if one of the suspect drugs is again clinically indicated.
- Antihistamines and corticosteroids form the cornerstone of treatment for most manifestations of allergic drug reaction.
- Follow established practice guidelines for treatment of anaphylaxis (see Chap. 13, Anaphylaxis), urticaria, angiodema (see Chap. 9, Urticaria and Angiodema), bronchospasm, and contact dermatitis (see Chap. 11, Allergic Contact Dermatitis).

Prevention

Prevention is the best strategy for avoiding drug reactions overall, especially for persons with a history of allergic drug reaction, as they are at increased risk for future hypersensitivity reactions. When possible, warn patients about drugs that cross-react with a drug known to have caused an adverse reaction, such as sulfa antibiotics and sulfonylureas.

There are four acceptable approaches to the patient with a history of immunologic drug reaction who requires retreatment with the same drug or class of drugs:

1. **Administer an alternate** (i.e., not cross-reactive) drug. Keep in mind that drug substitution may be costly both directly (increased acquisition cost) and indirectly (decreased efficacy and antibiotic resistance). It is important to review the chemical structure of the offending drug and to compare it to the proposed alternate drug. The absence of a reactive side chain is often all that is required for effective, safe substitution. For example, in the case of urticaria caused by captopril, either lisinopril or enalapril can be safely substituted, because these agents lack the sulfa-containing side chain found in captopril.
2. **Administer a potentially crossreactive drug under close medical supervision**, such as a cephalosporin in a patient with penicillin allergy. If available and reliable, skin testing can be performed before the drug is given to minimize the risk of anaphylaxis in patients giving a history compatible with immediate hypersensitivity. If the skin test is negative, the drug can be administered cautiously under close medical supervision. If the skin test is positive, a drug desensitization may be indicated.
3. **Provocative dose challenge** performed by an allergy consultant in the presence of resuscitative equipment can also be used to minimize risk. *Do not perform dose challenge with a potentially cross-reactive drug in a patient with a history of Stevens-Johnson syndrome or TEN [15].* In provocative dose challenge, a small initial test dose is selected and, if tolerated, doses are escalated until the full proposed thera-

TABLE 14-2. PRETREATMENT PROTOCOL FOR RADIOCONTRAST MEDIA

Time before the procedure (hr)	Drug and dose		
	Prednisone[a]	Cimetidine[b]	Diphenhydramine[c]
13	50 mg PO or IV	300 mg PO or IV	
7	50 mg PO or IV	300 mg PO or IV	
1	50 mg PO or IV	300 mg PO or IV	50 mg PO or IV

[a]Or methylprednisolone, 40 mg IV.
[b]Or ranitidine, 150 mg.
[c]Or chlorpheniramine, 10–12 mg.

peutic dose is attained. Challenge doses are administered 15–60 mins apart, depending on whether the drug is given parenterally or orally. It is important to use the same route of administration as will ultimately be used therapeutically.

4. **Pretreatment protocols** are available for some drugs to decrease the intensity of or prevent any non–IgE-mediated reaction that might occur. Table 14-2 outlines a sample protocol for patients with a history of radiocontrast media reactions.

5. **Perform desensitization** if no acceptable alternative drug exists. Desensitization applies only in circumstances in which type I hypersensitivity is known to be the mechanism behind the drug reaction, or in cases in which type I hypersensitivity could be operative but cannot be confirmed (e.g., lack of skin test for the drug). The goal is to slowly reintroduce a drug to which the patient is sensitive to prevent a life-threatening reaction. The drug is given every 15–30 mins in half-log$_{10}$ increments (approximately threefold) until a full therapeutic dose is achieved and tolerated without incident. The starting dose is typically determined by skin testing performed before desensitization—e.g., beginning with a dose equal to 1/100 of the dose producing a 5- to 8-mm wheal on skin testing. If the skin test is negative, start with 0.1 mL of a 1–3 μg/mL solution. A sample desensitization protocol for penicillin is given in Table 14-5. Important points concerning desensitization follow:

- Desensitization should only be performed under the supervision of a trained allergist in a location outfitted with resuscitation equipment for treating anaphylaxis. The patient will need secure, functioning IV access.
- The potential for reaction is diminished when oral formulations are used. If parenteral administration will ultimately be required, it is recommended that desensitization still be initiated with an oral agent and then repeated using the parenteral formulation.
- Beta-blockers should be withheld (taper if necessary) before procedure.
- The patient will remain desensitized only as long as the drug continues to be given. *Practically speaking, if the patient is without the drug for 24 hrs or more, desensitization will have to be performed again.*

6. Desensitization does not protect against the development of **mild skin reactions** such as urticaria or pruritus. It is possible to treat through these reactions without stopping the drug.

Special Topics

Penicillin Allergy
EPIDEMIOLOGY. As much as 10% of the general population claims to be allergic to penicillin. More than half report a history of rash. IgE-mediated reactions occur in

TABLE 14-3. PENICILLIN REACTIONS BY TIME COURSE

Immediate (<1 hr)	Accelerated (1–72 hrs)	Delayed (>72 hrs)
Anaphylaxis	Urticaria	Maculopapular rash
Urticaria	Bronchospasm	Fever
Angioedema	Erythema multiforme	Serum sickness
Bronchospasm	Maculopapular rash	Recurrent myalgias or urticaria
	Serum sickness	

about 2% of penicillin courses. Immediate (<1 hr) and accelerated reactions (1–72 hrs) occur at an incidence of about 0.3% each [16]. The estimated rate of anaphylaxis is 1/15,000 courses of therapy, or 0.007%. Penicillin is the most frequent known cause of anaphylaxis in humans. The highest rate of death is among adults aged 20–49.

CLASSIFICATION. Penicillin reactions are typically stratified by time course (Table 14-3). All immediate and many accelerated reactions are IgE-mediated.

CLINICAL MANIFESTATIONS. The most frequently reported sign of penicillin allergy is the maculopapular rash, occurring in 2–3% of courses. Urticaria, fever, and bronchospasm are the next most common reactions.

PATHOPHYSIOLOGY. Penicillin, like most commonly ingested drugs, is an LMW compound that requires conjugation with tissue proteins in order to elicit an allergic response. Approximately 93% of penicillin molecules are covalently bound to lysine residues in serum or cell-surface proteins, forming a penicilloyl moiety, referred to as the **major antigenic determinant**. All remaining penicillin conjugates (7%) are termed the **minor antigenic determinants**.

SKIN TESTING. Skin testing for penicillin hypersensitivity has been well studied and is both safe and reliable. It is still preferable, however, to administer an alternative agent to a patient with a sound history of penicillin hypersensitivity rather than to skin test that individual. *If no suitable alternative antibiotic can be substituted for penicillin, then skin testing is indicated.*

- The major antigenic determinant is available commercially as Pre-Pen for skin testing.
- The minor antigenic determinants are comprised of benzylpenicillin (or penicillin G), benzylpenicilloate, and benzylpenilloate, or a mixture of these. Only benzylpenicillin is available commercially in the United States. There is no standardized panel for the minor antigenic determinants, nor are they available as a RAST.
- The predictive value of the history of penicillin allergy in combination with skin testing in the assessment of penicillin hypersensitivity has been best studied in two large multicenter trials [17,18]. From these data, it can be predicted that 19% of patients with a positive history of penicillin allergy will have a positive skin test. Of note, however, is that 4–7% of patients with a negative history of penicillin allergy will also have a positive skin test. The incidence of reaction among skin test–negative subjects is less than 1% using a minor determinant mixture.

Important points to keep in mind concerning penicillin skin testing:

- Skin testing is not predictive of non–IgE-mediated reactions.
- The predictive value of skin testing with Pre-Pen and the minor determinants for reactivity to semi-synthetic penicillins is not known.

CROSS-REACTIVITY. Cross-reactivity among the beta-lactam antibiotics is variable, depending largely on the chemical structure of side-chains attached to the beta-lactam nucleus (Table 14-4). Most cephalosporin-specific IgE antibodies are directed against side-chain determinants, which rarely are homologous to semi-synthetic penicillin side chains. The complexity of the side chains increases with the generation of cephalosporin, so it follows that *cross-reactivity between third-generation cephalosporins*

TABLE 14-4. CROSS-REACTIVITY AMONG BETA-LACTAMS

Beta-lactam type	Degree of cross-reactivity with penicillin	Chemical structure
Semi-synthetic penicillins	High	
Cephalosporins	Low (8% or less)	
Carbapenems	High (approximately 45%)	
Monobactams	Trivial	

and penicillin is less than that between first- and second-generation cephalosporins and penicillin, except when side-chain similarities are present.

There is a paucity of data regarding cephalosporin and penicillin cross-reactivity. The best study, a compilation of case reports based on clinical history alone, estimated that 8% of patients with a history of penicillin allergy reacted to a cephalosporin [19]. The rate of reaction among patients without a history of penicillin allergy was 2%, approximating the baseline frequency of cephalosporin-induced skin reactions among all users. The monobactam aztreonam rarely cross-reacts with penicillin. However, aztreonam and ceftazidime share an identical side chain and are highly cross-reactive. The carbapenems (e.g., imipenem and meropenem) are highly cross-reactive with penicillin; 45% of patients with positive skin tests to penicillin react to one or more of imipenem determinants [20].

DESENSITIZATION. In situations in which a patient is skin test positive and there is no suitable alternative antibiotic, desensitization must be performed. A sample protocol follows (Table 14-5).

SULFONAMIDE ALLERGY

Sulfonamide antibiotics have a *p*-aminobenzoic acid ring, making them structurally similar to thiazide diuretics, furosemide, and sulfonylureas. This class of drugs is metabolized primarily by *N*-acetylation and secondarily by cytochrome P_{450} *N*-oxidation.

PATHOPHYSIOLOGY. Reactive oxygenated metabolites formed via the latter pathway combine avidly with tissue proteins to create an immunogen if not first detoxified by glutathione reductase. Genetically slow acetylators are more prone to allergic reactions, because they preferentially metabolize sulfonamide antibiotics via N-oxidation.

INCIDENCE. Overall, the incidence of allergic reactions to sulfonamides is high—approximately 2–10% (among patients not infected with HIV). *Adverse reactions to*

TABLE 14-5. PROTOCOL FOR ORAL PENICILLIN DESENSITIZATION

Time (min)	Units	Route
0	100	PO
15	200	PO
30	400	PO
45	800	PO
60	1,600	PO
75	3,200	PO
90	6,400	PO
105	12,500	PO
120	25,000	PO
135	50,000	PO
150	100,000	PO
165	200,000	PO
180	400,000	PO
195	50,000	SC
210	100,000	SC
225	200,000	SC
240	400,000	SC
255	800,000	SC
270	1,000,000	IM
285	100,000	IV
300	200,000	IV
315	400,000	IV

Modified from Sullivan TJ, Wedner HJ. Drug allergy. In: *Allergy theory and practice*, 2nd ed. Philadelphia: WB Saunders, 1992:548, with permission from Elsevier.

sulfonamides are 10–15 times more likely to occur in HIV-infected individuals than in the general population, because HIV-infected individuals have decreased levels of glutathione reductase [21].

CLINICAL MANIFESTATIONS. The most common manifestation of sulfonamide allergy is a maculopapular rash, occurring in an estimated 3% of users (compared to >50% of HIV-infected individuals). Urticaria, erythema multiforme, mucocutaneous reactions, and drug fever may also occur, but less frequently.

DIAGNOSIS. No reliable skin test reagent exists for sulfonamides.

DESENSITIZATION. Slow and rapid desensitization protocols have been devised for sulfonamide allergy; a rapid protocol is given in Table 14-6.

Local Anesthetics

Patients often report adverse reactions to local anesthetics (LAs), but rarely do these represent true allergy. LAs are often used in the settings of dental work or trauma, where vasovagal reactions or sympathetic stimulation from inadvertant IV injection of the anesthetic may be confused with anaphylaxis.

CLASSIFICATION. LAs are generally divided into two classes based on structure: *p*-aminobenzoic acid (PABA)-containing LAs (esters) and non–PABA-containing LAs (amides) (see Table 14-7). The PABA-containing LAs cross-react with one another. In contrast, the non–PABA-containing LAs are thought not to cross-react with each other or with the PABA-containing LAs.

TABLE 14-6. ORAL SULFONAMIDE DESENSITIZATION PROTOCOL (RAPID)

Steps	Concentration[a] (mg/mL)	Volume (mL)
Phase I: time interval between dosages is 15 mins		
1–4	0.000008/0.00004	0.5; 1; 2; 4
5–8	0.00008/0.0004	0.5; 1; 2; 4
9–12	0.0008/0.004	0.5; 1; 2; 4
13–16	0.008/0.04	0.5; 1; 2; 4
17–20	0.08/0.4	0.5; 1; 2; 4
21–24	0.8/4	0.5; 1; 2; 4
25	8/40	0.5
Phase II: time interval 30 mins between doses		
1	8/40	1
2	8/40	2
Phase III: time interval between doses		
1–4	8/40	2
5	8/40	3
6	8/40	5
7	8/40	8
8	8/40	10
9	80/400	1 tablet
10	80/400	Maintain with 1 tablet bid

[a]All dilutions made from stock solution of trimethoprim 40 mg + sulfamethoxazole 200 mg/5 mL.
Reprinted from Kalanadhabhatta V, Muppidi D, Sahni H, et al. Successful oral desensitization to trimethoprim-sulfamethoxazole in acquired immune deficiency syndrome. *Ann Allergy Asthma Immunol* 1996;77:394–400, with permission.

WORKUP. If the reported drug reaction has features compatible with hypersensitivity, and avoidance is not in the patient's best interest, proceed with epicutaneous skin testing using full-strength drug and positive and negative controls followed by intradermal testing with 0.02 mL of drug diluted 1:100 [22]. If skin testing is negative, proceed with SC incremental challenge using 0.1 mL of full-strength drug, graduating to 1 mL. It is important to note the following when assessing LA hypersensitivity:

- The reliability of skin testing for LAs has not been defined.
- It is best to choose a drug for skin testing and challenge that is not cross-reactive with the suspect drug; if the suspect drug is unknown, choose a non–PABA-contain-

TABLE 14-7. CLASSES OF LOCAL ANESTHETICS

PABA-containing	Non–PABA-containing
Chloroprocaine (Nesacaine)	Bupivacaine (Marcaine)
Procaine (Novocain)	Etidocaine (Duranest)
Tetracaine (Pontocaine)	Lidocaine (Xylocaine)
	Mepivacaine (Carbocaine)
	Prilocaine (Citanest)

ing LA (e.g., lidocaine) for testing. At Washington University, skin testing is performed using one PABA-containing LA (e.g., procaine or tetracaine) and two non–PABA-containing LAs (e.g., lidocaine and mepivacaine). It is wise to consult with the practitioner who desires to use the LA before skin testing, so that testing may be carried out with the LA of choice. If skin testing is negative, the LA that the practitioner (e.g., dentist) desires to use is selected for SC administration.

- Never use a preparation containing epinephrine or preservatives for skin testing. Epinephrine may cause a false-negative skin test, and parabens used as preservatives may cause a false-positive skin test.
- If the reported allergic reaction was delayed in onset, wait 24–48 hrs to confirm a negative skin test before proceeding to challenge, and wait 24–48 hrs after incremental challenge before proceeding to clinical use.
- Patients who have had a reaction to an LA should use preservative-free preparations in the future.

KEY POINTS

- Drug delivery (route, dose, timing) and host factors influence drug immunogenicity.
- Alterations in skin and mucous membranes are the most common manifestations of drug allergy.
- The predictive value of skin testing has been defined only for penicillin.
- Desensitization should only be performed under the supervision of a trained allergist in a location outfitted with resuscitation equipment.
- Cross-reactivity between penicillin and the newer generation cephalosporins is low.

REFERENCES

1. Faich GA. Adverse drug reaction monitoring. *N Engl J Med* 1986;314:1589–1592.
2. Porter J, Jick H. Drug-related deaths among medical inpatients. *JAMA* 1977; 237:879–881.
3. Armstrong B, Dinan B, Jick H. Fatal drug reactions in patients admitted to surgical services. *Am J Surg* 1976;132:643–645.
4. Anderson JA, Adkinson NF. Allergic reactions to drugs and biologic agents. *JAMA* 1987;258:2891–2899.
5. *Physicians' desk reference*. Montvale, NJ: Medical Economics Data, 2001.
6. Bianca M, Torres MJ, Garcia JJ, et al. Natural evolution of skin test sensitivity in patients allergic to beta-lactam antibiotics. *J Allergy Clin Immunol* 1999;103: 918–924.
7. Anonymous. Prospective study of ampicillin rash. Report of a Collaborative Study Group. *BMJ* 1973;844:7–9.
8. Tripathi A, Ditto AM, Grammer LC, et al. Corticosteroid therapy in an additional 13 cases of Stevens-Johnson syndrome: a total series of 67 cases. *Allergy Asthma Proc* 2000;21(2):101–105.
9. Roujeau JC, Kelly JP, Naldi L, et al. Medication use and the risk of Stevens-Johnson syndrome or toxic epidermal necrolysis. *N Engl J Med* 1995;333:1600–1607.
10. Mackowiak PA, LeMaistre CF. Drug fever: a critical appraisal of conventional concepts. *Ann Intern Med* 1987;106:728–733.
11. Lee WM. Drug-induced hepatotoxicity. *N Engl J Med* 1995;333:1118–1128.
12. Ditlove J, Weidmann P, Bernstein M, Massry SG. Methicillin nephritis. *Medicine* 1977;56(6):483–491.
13. Kancir LM, Tuazon CU, Cardella TA, Sheagren JN. Adverse reactions to methicillin and nafcillin during treatment of serious *Staphylococcus aureus* infections. *Arch Intern Med* 1978;138(6):909–911.
14. Weiss ME, Adkinson NF. Immediate hypersensitivity reactions to penicillin and related antibiotics. *Clin Allergy* 1988;18(6):515–540.
15. Vaillant L, Camenen I, Lorette G. Patch testing with carbamazepine: reinduction of an exfoliative dermatitis. *Arch Dermatol* 1989;125:299.

16. Task Force on Asthma and the Other Allergic Diseases. NIAID Task Force Report. Bethesda, MD: Department of Health, Education, and Welfare. NIH Publication 79-387/G, 1979.
17. Green GR, Rosenblum AH, Sweet LC. Evaluation of penicillin hypersensitivity: Value of clinical history and skin testing with penicilloyl-polylysine and penicillin G. *J Allergy Clin Immunol* 1977;60:339–345.
18. Sogn DD, Evans R, Shepherd GM et al. Results of the National Institute of Allergy and Infectious Diseases Collaborative Clinical Trial to test the predictive value of skin testing with major and minor penicillin derivatives in hospitalized adults. *Arch Intern Med* 1992;152:1025–1032.
19. Petz LD. Immunologic cross-reactivity between penicillins and cephalosporins: a review. *J Infect Dis* 1978;137:S74–S79.
20. Saxon A, Adelman DC, Patel A, et al. Imipenem cross-reactivity with penicillin in humans. *J Allergy Clin Immunol* 1988;82:213–217.
21. Beall G, Sanno M, Hussain H. Drug reactions and desensitization in AIDS. *Immunol Allergy Clin North Am* 1997;17:319–337.
22. DeShazo RD, Nelson HS. An approach to the patient with a history of local anesthetic hypersensitivity: experience with 90 patients. *Allergy Clin Immunol* 1979;63:387–394.

Insect Allergy

Khaled M. Abdel-Hamid

INTRODUCTION

Epidemiology

Prevalence of Insect Sting Allergy
In the general population, prevalence of reactions to bee stings is 0.3–3.0%. It is, however, as high as 20% among beekeepers.

Incidence of Anaphylaxis
A small number of sting allergy patients suffer from anaphylaxis during a sting challenge. Annually, 40–50 fatalities in the United States are attributed to insect sting anaphylaxis. This may be an underestimate, as anaphylactic reactions in predisposed individuals (especially the elderly) can result in myocardial infarction or cerebrovascular accidents that frequently end up being the presenting clinical diagnosis and eventual cause of death if fatality ensues.

Risk Factors for a Fatal Reaction
Risk factors for a fatal reaction include severe previous reaction (anaphylaxis), older age, significant cardiorespiratory disease, and medications (beta-blockers).

Entomology
Delivery of insect allergens can occur during insect **stinging** [e.g., bees, yellow jackets (YJs), hornets, wasps, fire ants, and harvester ants] or insect **biting** (e.g., mosquitoes, kissing bugs, deerflies). Stinging insects have been the most clinically important from the allergy perspective, although biting insects are slowly acquiring increasing importance.

Insects in the Hymenoptera (Latin for *membranous wings*) order deliver their venom using a modified ovipositor. Stings tend to cause **pain and not itching**. The ovipositor is avulsed from the insect in almost all cases involving bees and in 5–8% of YJ stings. The Hymenoptera order has three families of interest:

- Apidae family includes **honeybees and bumblebees**. These are docile insects that sting if provoked. Stings are mostly in farm areas, and exposure is frequently occupational. **Africanized honeybees** (killer bees, imported from Africa to Brazil 45 yrs ago) have reached the United States and are a problem in the southwest. These are very **aggressive** insects, and victims may suffer from **hundreds of stings**, with subsequent toxic reactions on initial exposure (see Toxic Reactions).
- Vespidae family includes **YJs, hornets, and wasps**. YJs are responsible for most of the reported insect allergy reactions. They are **aggressive** and attack without provocation. They nest in the ground and forage near garbage and around picnic areas. YJ nests can be disturbed by activities such as gardening and lawn mowing. Hornets are close relatives to YJs that nest in shrubs and can be disturbed during hedge clipping. Wasps, which are more common in Texas, tend to build their hives hanging from eaves and live in small groups; therefore, massive stinging is unlikely.

- Formicidae family includes **fire and harvester ants**, natives of South America. They are common in the eastern and central southern United States. They are the **non-winged** family of the order Hymenoptera. They characteristically attach themselves to the victim's skin using their jaws, then sting several times in a circular pattern, producing a characteristic **sterile pustule**.

In biting insect allergies, allergens are usually salivary proteins, and the bites frequently cause **itching and not pain**. Mosquitoes are rarely implicated in anaphylactic reactions, but they may cause large local reactions. Unlike mosquitoes, **deerfly and Triatoma** (kissing bug and bed bug) have been implicated in bite-induced **anaphylaxis**. The rest of this chapter focuses on reactions to Hymenoptera stings.

CAUSES

Pathophysiology

IgE-mediated reactions underlie the vast majority of allergic reactions to insect stings or bites.

Venom Biochemistry and Allergens

All the venom allergens are proteins, and many are enzymes. These include phospholipases (A, A_2, and C), hyaluronidase, melittin, and acid phosphates. Phospholipases tend to be antigenically less cross-reactive than hyaluronidases. Many other proteins and vasoactive amines are present in the venom. Smaller molecules, such as serotonin, histamine, dopamine, and kinin, have pharmacologic and toxic effects but do not induce IgE-mediated responses.

Local Reactions

Local reactions are classified by size (small and large) and latency (immediate and delayed). They manifest as swelling with localized pain and redness. Immediate (<4 hrs) and small reactions can be either IgE- or pharmacologically mediated. Larger as well as delayed reactions tend to be IgE mediated. Small reactions mostly disappear in a few hours, whereas larger reactions can peak in 24 hrs and last for 7–10 days. It is important to **distinguish large local reactions from systemic dermal** reactions. **Contiguity is the key feature** of a large local reaction (e.g., a finger is stung, and swelling spreads to include the whole extremity). If a finger is stung and a noncontiguous small reaction shows on the lip or chest, a **systemic dermal** reaction is the appropriate diagnosis. Be aware that large local reactions can be associated with **constitutional** manifestations such as malaise, fatigue, fever, and/or nausea.

Systemic Reactions

Systemic reactions are more serious and can be **limited** to dermal anaphylaxis (hives/urticaria and angioedema) or can **generalize** to involve the respiratory and cardiovascular systems with full-blown **anaphylaxis**. Occasionally, GI manifestations also occur.

Non-IgE Immune Reactions

Non-IgE immune reactions have been reported. **Serum sickness**–like response with fever, arthralgia, lymphadenopathy, and other symptoms can manifest 1–2 wks after insect sting. Serum sickness is mostly IgG mediated (although IgE may also contribute). **Neuritis, encephalitis, glomerulonephritis, and vasculitis** have all been reported in response to insect stings. Immune mechanisms other than type I reactions have been blamed for their pathogenesis.

Toxic Reactions

Venom is the insect's defense mechanism. It contains poisonous material in amounts that would not normally harm a big animal or human. Massive attacks (100s of stings) have been reported (Africanized honey bees, fire ants, and rarely with non-Africanized bees if their hives are disturbed). In these cases, large amounts of venom toxins are injected and may induce a toxic reaction that clinically simulates anaphylaxis and may end in death.

Differential Diagnosis

In addition to venom hypersensitivity, the following diagnoses should be considered:

- **Local reactions:** cellulitis, vasculitis, boils, and abscesses.
- **Systemic:** other causes of cardiorespiratory collapse such as vasovagal reaction, myocardial infarction, pulmonary embolism, sepsis, and other causes of anaphylaxis. In dermal anaphylaxis, do not forget to consider **drug reactions and food allergies**.

Natural History

Reactions to stinging insects tend to be stereotypical for the individual patient (i.e., the best predictor of the severity of a future reaction is the previous reaction).

Large local reactions recur in 80% of patients if they are stung again. Less than 5% of re-stinging, however, results in anaphylaxis.

Systemic reactions, on the other hand, are associated with 60% risk of anaphylaxis if the patient is re-challenged within the first few years, decreasing to 20% after 10 yrs without insect stings. This recurrence rate is significantly *lower in children*, especially with a history of previous isolated dermal anaphylaxis. **The early recurrence rate is nearly 80% in older patients with history of severe reaction in the past.** Multiple stings (simultaneously) and stings in close temporal proximity (within weeks) are also associated with increased risk of anaphylaxis.

Patients with history of serum sickness reaction or toxic reactions (after ≥ 100 stings) are at higher risk for sensitizations and future anaphylaxis.

The risk of future anaphylaxis and fatal outcome determines the need for venom immunotherapy.

PRESENTATION

History

Clinical data gathering aims at identifying the insect and the type of reaction (local vs systemic) and calculating the risk for future fatal reactions (medical comorbidities and medications). This information is critical for decision making about venom immunotherapy (VIT).

It is also important to gather details of the incident: location, activity that provoked the sting, type of insect, whether the stinger remained in the skin, how soon after the sting the reaction occurred (latency), how long the reaction lasted, previous sting incidents, significant medical problems after the sting (e.g., joint, kidney, neurologic).

Symptoms

- **Cutaneous:** pain, swelling (distribution, contiguity), flushing, urticaria and angioedema (lip, tongue, throat).
- **Respiratory and cardiovascular:** stridor, shortness of breath, wheezing, fainting, dizziness, palpitation, and cardiovascular collapse.
- **Gastrointestinal:** nausea, vomiting, abdominal cramps, and diarrhea.
- **Other:** malaise, fever, fatigue, skin rashes (vasculitis), joint pains, renal, mental or sensory complaints, etc.

Physical Exam

Primary doctors as well as emergency/urgent care physicians are more likely to see patients with physical findings. **The physical exam is usually negative** between episodes.

- **Cutaneous:** swelling, erythema, and angioedema.
- **Respiratory:** lip, tongue, or throat angioedema; stridor; wheezes; respiratory distress or failure. **Respiratory obstruction is the cause of death in 60% of fatalities.**
- **Cardiovascular:** tachycardia, flushing, hypotension, and vascular collapse/shock. 25% of the fatalities are due to cardiovascular collapse.
- Look for evidence of **infection** (more with wasps, as they tend to feed on infected decaying organic matter). This can manifest as cellulitis, abscesses, or even frank septicemia (the cause of 2% of insect sting–related deaths).

Remember that **most fatal reactions occur within 4 hrs** of the stinging incident. 10% of fatalities, however, are delayed (4–24 hrs).

MANAGEMENT

Workup

Skin Tests
Skin tests using purified venom (bee, YJ, hornet, and wasp) or whole body extract (fire ants) are the mainstay of diagnostic workup. After a major systemic reaction to suspected Hymenoptera sting, a 4- to 6-wk delay of skin testing is recommended to avoid a false-negative skin test during the post-anaphylaxis refractory period. Epicutaneous tests should precede intradermal tests to minimize risk of systemic reactions in highly sensitive individuals. A maximum extract concentration of 1 μg/mL is used, with sensitivity of 90–95%. This concentration unfortunately may result in 20% false-positive results. Lower concentrations, however, are associated with an unacceptable sensitivity of <70%.

Practically, a patient with suspected insect sting allergy is tested for **all** stinging insects, even if the history may suggest that a particular insect is the likely culprit. This is justified by the life-threatening nature of the disease and possible fatal sequelae if the diagnosis is missed. **Cross-reactivity** of skin testing has been observed within the vespid family (YJs closer to hornets, whereas wasps are much less likely to cross-react). Honeybee skin test detects honeybee allergy and is likely to be positive in bumblebee allergy as well. **Vespids do not cross-react with bees.** Although the question of "cross-reactivity vs multiple hypersensitivity" can be resolved using RAST inhibition assays, this is seldom needed or used in clinical practice.

Radioallergosorbent Test
RAST is 80% sensitive compared to skin tests but detects an additional 10% of patients that are allergic with negative skin tests. **Both tests are required if the history suggests sting allergy and skin tests are negative or contraindicated.**

Severity of the reaction and the risk of future anaphylaxis do not correlate with the intensity of the local reaction to skin test or to the RAST titer.

Sting Challenge
Sting challenge in the ICU setting is **not** used for diagnostic purposes.

Treatment

Immediate
If the stinger is still in the skin it should be removed immediately (without squeezing). However, stinger removal is only useful in the first 3–5 mins after stinging. After that time, the stinger has usually emptied its contents in the sting site.

- **Small local reactions (<2-in. diameter):** Do not usually require treatment, but ASA and cold compresses may provide symptomatic relief.
- **Larger local reactions (>2-in. diameter):** May last up to 7–10 days and will benefit from antihistamine, analgesics, cold compresses, and, if symptoms are severe or

constitutional, a 2- to 3-day course of moderate doses of prednisone (e.g., 40 mg/day for an average adult).

- **Systemic reaction and anaphylaxis:** Treated according to standard protocols for respiratory and circulatory collapse (see Chap. 4, Asthma, and Chap. 13, Anaphylaxis, for details).

Long-Term Management: Avoidance and Prophylaxis for Sensitive Individuals

- Carry an **anaphylaxis kit** (e.g., Ana-Kit or EpiPen) at all times. Use the kit as soon you are stung, without waiting for a reaction to manifest. Go immediately to the ER for evaluation and observation if you needed to use the anaphylaxis kit. Call 911 and don't drive to the ER.
- Avoid wearing bright colors or scents, which may attract insects.
- **Wear gloves** while working in the garden.
- Get professional help for eradication of Hymenoptera nests if necessary at your house or backyard.
- Carry special Hymenoptera insecticide spray.
- Avoid drinking from **unattended open soda cans** (insects may have been trapped inside the can).
- Wear long **protective clothes** in grass fields and avoid loose fitting clothes that may trap insects within.
- Wear a **Medic-Alert bracelet**. Avoid being alone in situations where you may be stung. Inform people with you of your condition and what to do if you are stung.

Special Considerations

Venom Immunotherapy

VIT is the standard of care for selected insect allergy patients.

INDICATIONS AND PATIENT SELECTION. The decision to start an allergic patient on immunotherapy should be individualized, taking into consideration his or her risk factors, coexisting medical conditions, medications, and lifestyle. **It should only be considered in skin test– and/or RAST-positive patients with history of reaction to Hymenoptera stings.** General guidelines are listed in Table 15-1.

VENOM SELECTION. The common practice is to treat patients using all the venoms to which the patient reacts. If definite identification of the culprit insect (e.g., YJ) is possible, and the patient has a mildly positive skin reaction to a known cross-reacting venom (e.g., paper wasp), it is possible to eliminate the cross-reacting venom from the VIT protocol (with reduced cost and potential side effects). The decision is individualized, and an experienced allergist should weigh the risks and benefits.

TABLE 15-1. GENERAL GUIDELINES FOR VENOM IMMUNOTHERAPY (VIT)

Reaction	Is VIT indicated?
Local reaction (small or extensive)	No
Anaphylaxis	
Mild/dermal in children	No
Mild/dermal in adults	Yes
Moderate or severe	Yes
Serum sickness	Yes
Toxic reactions	Yes

Note: Progressively larger local reactions in high-risk adults (e.g., beekeepers may warrant initiation of VIT).

DOSING SCHEDULES. **VIT injection should be administered only in a medical facility** staffed and equipped to manage possible adverse reaction including anaphylaxis. Traditional VIT is initiated at 0.01–0.1 μg (depending on **intensity of the skin reaction** to epicutaneous and intradermal tests and **not on severity of the sting reaction**). The dose is increased on a weekly basis to the maintenance dose. Once maintenance dose is reached, dosing should be done every 4 wks in the first year, 6 wks in the second year, and possibly every 8 wks in the third year and onward.

Under close supervision, protocols exist for **rapid escalation** of the dose to achieve the maintenance dose over a shorter period of time—2 wks instead of 11 wks **(rush)** or even over only 3 days (ultrarush).

For **maintenance**, the target dose is usually 100 μg of each venom (or 300 μg of the mixed vespid venom containing equal amounts of YJ, yellow hornet, and white-faced hornet venom). Some studies suggest that the honeybee target dose should be higher (150–200 μg), as the traditional maintenance dose is associated with 80% protection rate only.

REACTIONS TO VIT. **VIT reactions are commonly local** in nature. Splitting the dose (i.e., over 2 injection sites) may solve the problem. In persistent large local reactions, co-injection of small amounts of epinephrine or steroids may resolve the problem. One study suggested that routine use of oral antihistamines might both reduce the incidence of local and systemic reactions and enhance the efficacy of VIT.

Systemic reactions during VIT are less common than local reactions, with an incidence of 3–12% per patient and with no reported fatalities over two decades. However, systemic reactions require reviewing the injection protocol carefully. Usually, subsequent doses are reduced to one-third or one-fourth the dose that caused the reaction, and smaller escalation steps are used until the maintenance dose is reached.

Remember that unlike reactions to aeroallergen immunotherapy, which may be controlled by reducing the maintenance dose, **VIT efficacy (which is a matter of life and death) requires a certain maintenance dose to be achieved.** The vast majority of patients are able to tolerate the dose necessary to achieve protection.

PREGNANCY AND VIT. VIT has been found to be safe during pregnancy. Initiation of VIT and dose escalation are, however, not routinely recommended during pregnancy for fear of the effect of systemic reactions on the fetus. However, in high-risk individuals, the small risk of VIT-induced systemic reactions (occurring in a medical facility where the VIT is administered) should be weighed against the benefits of protection against possible sting-induced anaphylaxis during pregnancy.

TREATMENT FAILURES. Treatment failures are very rare. **Review and repeat skin test** for errors in venom selection, or **aim for higher maintenance doses** if needed (especially with honeybees).

CESSATION OF VIT AND EFFICACY MONITORING. After 3 years of VIT, protective efficacy reaches a level of $\geq$ 98% for vespids (80–85% for honeybees). Some authors feel there is no need to monitor patients for protection given the consistently high level of success of VIT reported in the literature. Others suggest that a follow-up **skin test every 1–2 yrs** might detect the 20% of VIT patients who convert to a negative skin test during the course of therapy. If this conversion occurs, VIT can safely be discontinued; otherwise, VIT should **continue for 3–5 yrs**. Rarely, some patients may need to continue forever on VIT if sting reactions occur while on adequate maintenance dose (albeit milder than their initial pre-VIT reactions), or if VIT-induced reactions preclude escalation to maintenance dose. Some experts advocate **>5 yrs (or even lifelong)** VIT for patients with initial near-fatal anaphylaxis. Using specific anti-venom IgG level as a criterion to discontinue VIT has not been widely accepted.

Fire Ants

Fire ants (*Solenopsis invecta* and *Solenopsis richteri*) are responsible for an increasing number of insect hypersensitivity reactions. Although they are more common in the southeast and south-central states, they are spreading both westward and northward. In addition to local and systemic reactions, they also cause a characteristic **sterile pustule** within 24 hrs at injection site. These pustules are caused by the very high **alkaloid** content in their venom and are **not IgE mediated**.

Diagnosis and treatment of fire ant sting hypersensitivity follow the same guidelines as for other Hymenoptera families. The notable difference, however, is that only whole body extract (WBE), and not purified venom, is available for skin testing and immunotherapy. However, **Solenopsis WBE**, unlike Hymenoptera WBE, has **proved effective** for immunotherapy, because it contains the major *Solenopsis* allergens.

KEY POINTS

* **Fifty cases of fatal anaphylaxis** resulting from insect sting allergy are reported annually in the United States. **Respiratory obstruction is the cause of death in 60% of cases.**
* Insect sting allergy is an **IgE-mediated immediate hypersensitivity** reaction to proteins in insect venom. Reaction **severity tends to be stereotypic** for the patient.
* VIT is a **standardized** therapeutic modality that reduces significantly the risk of future life-threatening anaphylactic reactions.
* **The risk of future anaphylaxis determines the need for VIT.**
* Skin tests for sting allergy are **more sensitive** than RAST tests.
* Skin test results should be interpreted in the context of clinical history and the **understanding of the allergen cross-reactivity patterns**.
* **Stinging insect avoidance measures, anaphylaxis kits, and Medic-Alert bracelets** are integral parts of the management of sting allergy.

SUGGESTED READING

Afrasiabi R. Insect allergy. In: Nagua SM, Gershwin ME, eds. *Allergy and immunology secrets*. Philadelphia: Hanley & Belfus, 2001;175–84.

Graft Df, Golden DBK, Reismean R, et al. The discontinuation of *Hymenoptera* venom immunotherapy: position statement. *J Allergy Clin Immunol* 1998;101(5):573–575.

Levine MI, Lockey RF, eds. *Monograph on insect allergy*, 3rd ed. Milwaukee: American Academy of Allergy and Immunology, 1995.

Reisman RE. Insect sting allergy. In: Lieberman P, Anderson J, eds. *Current clinical practice: allergic diseases: diagnosis and treatment*, 2nd ed. Totowa, NJ: Humana Press, 2000;73–83.

Yunginger JW. Insect allergy. In: Middleton E Jr, Reed CE, et al., eds. *Allergy principles and practice*, 5th ed. St. Louis: Mosby, 1998;1063–1072.

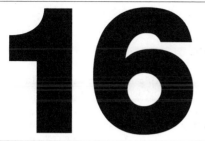

Food Allergy and Other Adverse Food Reactions

Khaled M. Abdel-Hamid

INTRODUCTION

Definition and Classification

Food allergy refers to a small group of **adverse food reactions (AFRs)** for which an immunologic mechanism has been identified. The vast majority of these are IgE-mediated (Gell and Coombs classification type I) with immediate postingestion manifestations (minutes to hours), though in few cases other immune mechanisms have been postulated with signs and symptoms manifesting over hours to days. The more inclusive term *adverse food reactions* includes food intolerance.

Etiology

AFRs can be etiologically classified as food toxicity, poisoning, idiosyncrasy, and pharmacologic reactions. In a minority of cases, food additives (preservatives and food colors) have been implicated in AFRs. In many cases, suspected AFR should be confirmed using **double-blind, placebo-controlled food challenge (DBPCFC)**, which is the **gold standard** for establishing the diagnosis of AFR.

Epidemiology

Prevalence of Adverse Food Reactions
Nearly 20–25% of parents believe their children suffer from food allergies justifying modification of their diets. Studies of oral food challenge, however, suggest that only 8% of children ≤ 3 yrs can be labeled as having a food allergy. The percentage of children affected decreases with age, and by adulthood, the prevalence of food allergies is 1.5%. Cow's milk allergy affects 2.5% of children in the first 2 yrs of life, whereas egg and peanut allergy have prevalences of 1.5% and 0.5%, respectively. Food allergy is more prevalent in patients with atopy. 30% of children with severe atopic dermatitis (AD) and 10% of those with asthma are found to have food allergies.

Incidence of Food Anaphylaxis
Food is postulated to be a major cause of systemic anaphylaxis and anaphylactoid reactions, with an annual incidence of four cases per million population and an estimated 500 deaths annually.

Foods Commonly Incriminated
Although any food can cause food allergy, only a few foods are believed to cause >90% of clinically significant cases. In children, cow's milk, wheat, soybeans, eggs, and peanuts are the most common offenders. Peanuts, tree nuts, and crustaceans are the foods likely to be involved in food allergies in adults and are the foods most likely to cause food-induced anaphylaxis.

CAUSES

Pathophysiology

Food Allergens

Major food allergens tend to be glycoproteins with a molecular weight of 10–70 kd that tend to be heat stable and withstand cooking, food processing, and enzymatic proteolysis after ingestion.

Cross-Reactivity in Food Allergy

Skin testing and *in vitro* radioallergosorbant (RAST) tests demonstrate cross-reactivity within different food families (e.g., peanuts and peas are both in the legume family). This cross-reactivity is usually of no clinical significance, and patients tend to react clinically to a single food (e.g., peanuts and not peas) despite multiple positive skin tests and RAST results. These results should thus be interpreted in the context of clinical presentation.

Clinical cross-reactivity, however, is present in an interesting IgE-mediated reaction known as the **oral allergy syndrome (OAS)**. In OAS, patients with aeroallergen hypersensitivity (to pollens, grass, etc.) may develop oral symptoms (labial pruritus, perioral urticarial rash, etc.) on consumption of certain fresh fruits and vegetables. Cross-reacting allergens involved in OAS are minor antigens that are **heat labile** and are destroyed by cooking and food processing.

GI Defense Mechanisms

The GI mucosa is the first-line barrier between the body and foreign food proteins. More than 98% of ingested proteins are broken down to simple nonimmunogenic units (amino acids and oligopeptides) by proteolysis. However, traces of food proteins are absorbed as **intact antigens**, with consequent development of tolerance to these antigens. The mechanism of tolerance is not completely understood, but it involves both B and T lymphocytes with clonal deletion, anergy, and/or active suppression. GI defense mechanisms mature with age and are possibly enhanced by factors such as consumption of breast milk early in life. This may explain the higher incidence of food allergy in infants compared with adults and the protective role of exclusive breast-feeding in the first year of life.

Natural History

Food allergies are more frequently encountered in **children**, possibly because of immaturity of GI defense mechanisms and/or immaturity of the immune system. As children with food allergy, confirmed by DBPCFC, get older, they outgrow certain food allergies (e.g., to milk, eggs, and wheat, but **not** to crustaceans or peanuts). Frequently, their skin tests and RAST assays remain positive despite a negative food challenge. **Strict elimination of allergens from the diet increases the probability that food allergies will resolve** (nearly one-third of children and adults lose clinical reactivity after 1–2 yrs of allergen avoidance). Prevalence of positive food challenges drops from 8% in children (≤ 3 yrs) to approximately 1.5% in adults.

It is unfortunate, however, that loss of reactivity is food-specific, and that foods associated with most fatal anaphylaxis (peanuts, tree nuts, crustaceans, and fish) are associated with life-long clinical reactivity despite strict elimination.

Infants with non–IgE-mediated food intolerance also respond favorably to allergen avoidance with long-term loss of clinical reactivity. **Celiac disease**, unfortunately, is an exception, and life-long avoidance of gluten is mandatory for disease control.

PRESENTATION

Types of Food Reactions and Clinical Presentation

IgE-Mediated Immune Reactions to Food

IgE-mediated immune reactions comprise almost all food allergies. Previous exposure to allergenic food, usually intermittently, is required for the development of this type of immune reaction. Antigen-specific IgE attaches to high-affinity IgE receptors on mast cells and basophils where, on binding to their specific allergens, they trigger the process of mast cell (and basophil) activation and degranulation with the release of cytokines and other mediators. Early-phase reactions develop within minutes and frequently are followed by a late-phase reaction a few hours later.

Clinical syndromes associated with type I hypersensitivity reactions range from urticarial rashes (±angioedema) and OAS (see Cross-Reactivity in Food Allergy) to full-blown systemic anaphylaxis with vascular collapse. Systemic anaphylaxis usually starts within a few minutes to an hour after food ingestion. Occasionally, mild oral or skin symptoms may be a prelude to fatal anaphylaxis. Late-onset anaphylaxis almost never starts more than 4 hrs after allergen ingestion.

With more prolonged exposure to an allergenic food, allergic rhinoconjunctivitis and bronchial asthma may manifest, especially in patients with AD.

In a few cases, IgE-mediated food allergy can present as infantile colic, eosinophilic gastroenteritis, and infantile gastroesophageal reflux disease. Diagnosis of the latter group requires a high index of suspicion and endoscopic biopsy.

Food-associated exercise-induced anaphylaxis is a recently established class of food allergy. In this interesting disease, anaphylaxis occurs only if vigorous exercise occurs 1–2 hrs after ingestion of certain foods (or less commonly any food).

Non–IgE-Mediated Immune Reactions to Food

Types II and III of non–IgE-mediated immune reactions as well as cell-mediated food reactions have been implicated in rare cases of AFRs.

Food-induced thrombocytopenia (type II reaction to cow's milk) has been reported (but is exceedingly rare).

A rare syndrome known as *Heiner's syndrome*, first described in 1956, is believed to result from hypersensitivity to cow's milk. Early aspiration and sequestration of milk in the lungs initiates an immune reaction manifesting as a pneumonia-like disease with pulmonary infiltrates associated with iron-deficiency anemia and pulmonary hemosiderosis. In addition to IgE, patient's serum contains high levels of a precipitating IgG antibody to cow's milk. Disease pathology is likely mediated via immune complex and cell-mediated hypersensitivity-type reactions. This rare disease has also been described in breast-fed infants.

Celiac disease, or gluten enteropathy, is possibly mediated in part by a type IV hypersensitivity to gluten in addition to direct gluten toxicity.

Nonimmunologic Reactions to Food

A variety of mechanisms are involved in several AFRs.

Scombroid fish poisoning is an anaphylactoid type reaction resulting from the action of bacterial decarboxylase on histidine-rich fish meat (tuna, mackerel, bonito, mahi mahi). Histamine is generated enzymatically, and when the fish is ingested, the patient complains of burning mouth sensation, pruritus, flushing, nausea, vomiting, headache, and even vascular collapse.

Similar symptoms can occur as a result of ingestion of histamine-rich foods such as Roquefort and Parmesan cheeses, eggplant, spinach, and red wine. Ingestion of foods rich in serotonin (tomato, pineapple, avocado, and banana) or tyramine (cheese and wine) can be associated with **"pharmacologic"** symptoms such as flushing, headaches, and palpitation. These symptoms are much more pronounced in individuals on MAOIs.

Idiosyncratic intolerance is exemplified by lactose intolerance, which is frequently indistinguishable from GI presentations of IgE-mediated milk allergy. Careful history taking usually resolves the confusion. Asian, Arab, or black ethnic background; later age of onset (over 7 yrs); and occasional association with recent gastroenteritis are associated with lactose intolerance.

Several food-induced GI syndromes are identified that are similar to IgE-mediated syndromes with no evidence of food-specific IgE. These include: gastroenteritis, proctocolitis, enteropathy (e.g., gluten enteropathy), and gastroesophageal reflux disease. Gluten enteropathy is frequently associated with an intensely pruritic vesicular condition known as *dermatitis herpetiformis*, which affects extensor surfaces and buttocks.

Food-induced migraine is a poorly understood entity that has been reported in some patients with positive DBPCFC. The mechanism is unknown.

MANAGEMENT

Workup

History
Careful history taking is the most powerful diagnostic tool for food allergies. In many cases, physical exam is completely normal and the patient (or family) frequently seeks medical advice for confirmation of a suspected food-induced reaction. A detailed history of previous or current episodes of AFR should include the following:

- Food(s) suspected of provoking the reaction.
- Description of the reaction: age of onset of first reaction, latency between ingestion and onset of symptoms, rate of progression of the reaction, duration of the reaction, course (i.e., intermittent or chronic), reproducibility and similar episodes in response to other foods or same food in a different form (raw, cooked, or canned), associated events (e.g., exercise, alcohol consumption), how long since last episode.
- Systemic manifestations of the reaction:

  - Cutaneous: hives, pruritus, swelling, flushing
  - Oral: pruritus; lip, tongue, or throat swelling; difficulty swallowing; change of voice
  - Respiratory: difficulty breathing, stridor, wheezing, cough
  - GI: nausea, vomiting, abdominal pain/colic, bloating, diarrhea, bloody stool
  - Cardiovascular: dizziness, palpitations, collapse
  - General: headaches, history of malabsorption, chronic weight loss, delayed developmental milestones, chronic anemia

- Severity of the reaction and the need for medical attention (e.g., no treatment needed, phoned or visited primary care physician, ER visit or hospital admission, and nature of treatment received).
- Past medical history: allergic rhinitis/conjunctivitis, bronchial asthma; exacerbation of symptoms with food ingestion.
- Family history of atopic diseases.

Physical Exam
Physical exam is frequently negative.

In emergency situations, ascertain the cardiovascular and respiratory condition of the patient to rule out anaphylaxis.

If in doubt about the etiology in a patient with cardiovascular collapse and suspicious history or suggestive signs (e.g., hives, wheezes in patient without history of bronchial asthma, protracted or nonresponsive shock state), consider and possibly treat as anaphylaxis. Obtain blood for serum tryptase level (within 4 hrs) for later confirmation.

In nonemergency situations (e.g., elective office visit), look for the following signs:

- Cutaneous: urticaria, angioedema, AD/eczema, dermatitis herpetiformis
- Respiratory: distress, wheezing
- Evidence of upper respiratory allergies (e.g., pale enlarged nasal turbinates, postnasal drip, pharyngeal cobblestoning, and pretonsillar throat erythema)
- General: dehydration, anemia, malnutrition, failure to thrive (in children)

Food Diaries
Ask the patient to prospectively keep a detailed listing of all ingested foods (and medications) and any AFR and AFR-associated events (e.g., exercise) for a few weeks. This is most useful if manifestations are intermittent. It is also more objective than relying on the patient's recollection of previous events. Analysis of food diaries often reveals unexpected associations and helps to interpret skin tests and RAST assays in the proper context.

Diet Elimination

This technique is useful in chronic nonintermittent manifestations of suspected food allergies. It involves switching the patient to a diet consisting of foods believed to be the least allergenic in most people (e.g., rice and lamb). Resolution of symptoms suggests a food-related etiology. Reintroduction of selected foods over time (one new food item every 3–4 days) may help identify culprit foods. This approach is contraindicated in suspected food-induced anaphylaxis. Care should be taken to avoid malnutrition, vitamin deficiencies, and dehydration.

Skin Tests

Skin prick tests (SPTs) are safe except in patients with a reliable history of near fatal anaphylaxis. A positive test is very specific but has a poor positive predictive value (50% in children and 5% or less in adults). Thus, avoid using SPTs out of clinical context. A negative SPT, however, rules out IgE-mediated food allergy (negative predictive value near 100%). Intradermal skin tests have no role in diagnosis of food allergies. If suspected food allergy is associated with fresh and raw fruits or vegetables (e.g., OAS), then the prick-and-prick technique is used: A fresh food is peeled and pricked by SPT device, followed by pricking the patient's skin.

RAST and Other Lab Investigations

RAST measures levels of food-specific IgE in the serum. These usually have only 80% of the sensitivity of SPTs and are more expensive, and the results are not immediately available. Order RAST testing only if SPTs cannot be performed (e.g., diffuse chronic skin disease, patient cannot stop antihistamines), produce results that are inconsistent with clinical history or are contraindicated. Recent studies have suggested some utility for **capture allergen protein RAST** (CAP-RAST, a more sensitive RAST test but with more false-positive results) in determining the level of risk of oral food challenges. This "risk stratification" can then be used to decide whether food challenge is contraindicated, should be done in a medical facility, or can be performed at home.

Food Challenges

DBPCFC is the gold standard for diagnosing AFR and is usually performed by an allergist/immunologist familiar with the management of anaphylaxis. A positive challenge does not necessarily identify the mechanism of the reaction (IgE-, non–IgE-, or non–immune-mediated reaction). **Food challenges are contraindicated in suspected food-induced anaphylaxis.** Good history and consistent SPT are usually sufficient to establish a diagnosis without a food challenge. With vague history and inconclusive SPT, an open challenge may be indicated, followed, if positive, by a blinded challenge. Details of food-challenge techniques are available in standard allergy textbooks.

Other Tests

Other tests may be indicated for the diagnosis of AFR (immune and nonimmune). Serum tryptase levels are useful in some cases of food-induced anaphylaxis if serum is collected early after the event (1–2 hrs, but may be useful up to 6 hrs after anaphylaxis). CBC with differential counts in suspected chronic allergies and atopy (eosinophilia) or anemia associated with AFR (celiac disease and Heiner's syndrome). Hydrogen breath tests can confirm lactose intolerance, and endoscopic biopsies are required to establish the diagnosis of eosinophilic syndrome of the GI tract.

Treatment

Acute reactions presenting to the ER should be treated immediately and aggressively (see Chap. 13, Anaphylaxis). Other causes of collapse and shock should not be ignored either. If food ingestion is recent, gastric lavage may help reduce allergen load. Oropharyngeal laryngeal angioedema may benefit from aerosolized epinephrine and may require endotracheal intubation. **All treated cases should be observed for a minimum of 4 hrs** (preferably 8–10 hrs, and for up to 24 hrs in the case of severe reactions) in the ER before discharge with referral to an allergist/immunologist.

The **only long-term control measure for food allergy is strict elimination from the diet**. In children, but not adults, many foods can be reintroduced after a few years of elimination without reactivation of allergic reactions. With certain foods, such as peanuts (see Natural History), however, life-long elimination is required. **Patient education** is the most important component of the management plan. The patient's family and caregivers of young children and infants also need education. This includes careful checking of food labels, education about alternative food names and "hidden" foods (e.g., casein for milk), heightened awareness in restaurants (only the cook knows!), and elimination of foods with unidentified ingredients. Avoiding situations where cross-contamination of foods is frequent (e.g., open buffets and salad bars) may make the difference between life and death in patients with history of food-induced anaphylaxis.

History of anaphylaxis or other IgE-mediated reactions warrants the prescription of preloaded epinephrine kits (e.g., Ana-Kit, EpiPen, and EpiPen Jr autoinjectors). **Dual** packs are recommended to avoid the risk of injector malfunctions and recurrence of symptoms before arrival to a medical facility. Thorough education of the patient, family, and care providers is necessary. **Emphasize the absolute need to have injectable epinephrine within reach at all times (no exceptions)**. The prescription should be refilled every 6 mos, and the kit should be protected from extreme temperature (avoid automobile glove compartments or freezing weather). The patient should use epinephrine at the earliest sign or symptoms of a reaction. The patient should also be instructed to call 911 to be transported to the ER (and not to drive him- or herself) as soon as the epinephrine is administered, regardless of how good he or she feels. Risk factors for fatal anaphylaxis include poorly controlled bronchial asthma, older age with compromised cardiovascular health, use of beta-adrenergic blockers, being away from home, and a delay of epinephrine injection >1 hr after appearance of symptoms. **Patients should wear a medical alert bracelet all the time**.

Children with milk allergy can be managed with formula substitutes: soy-based (e.g., Isomil, ProSoyBee), casein protein hydrolysate (e.g., Nutramigen, Carnation Good Start) or, in cases of extreme intolerance, elemental amino acid–based formula (Neocate).

Antihistamines, cromolyn, corticosteroids, and ketotifen (not available in the United States) are of no proven value in long-term management of food allergies. Immunotherapy with food antigens has not been proved beneficial and are likely to be unacceptably risky.

Recent studies evaluating the benefits of maternal avoidance of allergenic foods during the last trimester of pregnancy and during lactation, as well as exclusive breast-feeding in the first year of life, remain to be validated.

Further patient information and support can be obtained from Food Allergy Network, Fairfax, VA (phone: 1-800-929-4040; Web address: www.foodallergy.org).

Special Topics

Allergies to Food Additives

Over the years, many case reports have blamed **food dyes, preservatives, and additives**, such as aspartame and monosodium glutamate (MSG), for a variety of allergic or pseudoallergic reactions. Reactions range from acute or chronic urticaria and induction or exacerbation of bronchial asthma to migraine headaches and behavioral disorders, such as hyperactivity and attention deficit disorders. Larger-scale trials and DBPCFC have not substantiated most of these associations.

MSG was reported to cause the "Chinese restaurant syndrome" rarely in individuals consuming large amounts of MSG. Symptoms start 30 mins after ingestion and manifest with anxiety, headache, sweating, flushing, palpitation, tightness, a burning sensation in the face and chest, and a crawling sensation of the skin. The condition is self-limited and subsides over 1–2 hrs.

Food preservatives, such as benzoate, butylated hydroxyzole, and butylated hydroxytoluene, were not associated with AFR in well-designed studies. Sulfites, on the other hand, were found to exacerbate asthma in a small percentage of asthmatics (<5%), particularly in patients with severe asthma. The mechanism behind the reaction is not clear, but the exposure occurs in part by inhalation of SO_2 gas that evolves from metabisulfite-preserved foods (especially at salad bars) during ingestion. Certain individuals with inherent sulfite oxidase deficiency may be more at risk for AFR.

In European studies, artificial food colors have been blamed for ≥ 15% of chronic urticaria cases, whereas in the Unites States this high percentage has never been substantiated. Tartrazine (food dye yellow #5) has been reported to cross-react with aspirin in aspirin-sensitive asthmatics, a finding that could not be validated in DBPCFC in aspirin-sensitive individuals. However, yellow #5 is implicated in rare cases of asthma independent of aspirin.

The sugar substitute aspartame has been implicated in very few cases of chronic urticaria. A multi-center study using DBPCFC was unable to confirm this association. *Sugar allergy*, a term coined in the mid-1980s, was believed to contribute to attention deficit disorder and juvenile delinquency behavior, an assumption completely refuted by controlled studies.

In summary, food additives' role in AFR is more anecdotal than factual. **Food additives available on the market at the present time contribute very little, if at all, to allergic food reactions.**

KEY POINTS

- More patients believe they have food allergies than what could be found using blinded food challenges.
- Food "allergy" is a subset of a larger group of **adverse food reactions (AFRs)**. AFRs include idiosyncratic, toxic, and pharmacologic, as well as allergic, reactions to food.
- **Young children** have more food allergies than adults but tend to **outgrow** their allergies, especially after a period of strict elimination.
- **Milk, egg, wheat, soybean, and peanut cause more than 90%** of food allergies in children.
- **Oral allergy syndrome** results from cross-reactivity of food allergen with certain pollen aeroallergens.
- **Detailed history and skin tests are the most valuable diagnostic tools** of food allergies.
- There is **no role for immunotherapy** in the treatment of food allergy.
- **Patient (and parent) education and anaphylaxis kits** are the most powerful life-saving measures in severe food allergy.

SUGGESTED READING

Anderson, J. Food allergy and intolerance. In: Lieberman P, Anderson J, eds. *Current clinical practice: allergic diseases: diagnosis and treatment*, 2nd ed. Totowa, NJ: Humana Press, 2000;283–302.

Ditto AM, Grammer LC. Food allergy. In: Patterson R, Grammer LC, Greenberger PA, eds. *Allergic diseases diagnosis and management*, 5th ed. Philadelphia: Lippincott Williams & Wilkins, 1997;285–304.

Sampson HA. Food allergy. In: Baker J, ed. *JAMA Primer on allergic and immunologic diseases*, 4th ed. Chicago: America Medical Association, 1997;1888–1895.

Sicherer SH. Manifestations of food allergy: evaluation and management. *Am Fam Physician* 1999;59(2):415–430.

Teuber, SS. Food allergy and intolerance. In: Nagua SM, Gershwin ME, eds. *Allergy and immunology secrets*. Philadelphia: Hanley & Belfus, 2001;159–176.

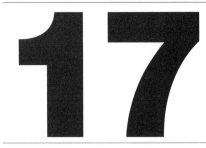

Latex Allergy

Alpa L. Jani

INTRODUCTION

Most strictly, *latex allergy* (LA) refers to an immediate hypersensitivity reaction caused by exposure to products containing natural rubber latex in persons with latex-specific IgE [1]. Operationally, the term sometimes includes patients with latex-specific IgE or clinical history alone. Patients whose symptoms are limited to contact dermatitis occurring through a delayed hypersensitivity mechanism or limited to a nonimmunologic, irritant contact dermatitis should more appropriately be identified as latex sensitive.

Manufacture of latex products begins with collection of the milky sap of the rubber tree *Hevea brasiliensis* into cups of ammonia. Accelerators, antioxidants, and preservatives are then added. Dipped latex products, such as gloves, are thought to carry the highest allergen content and are the cause of most anaphylactic reactions to natural rubber latex [2]. Cornstarch applied to gloves for lubrication adsorbs allergenic proteins, allowing increased transference to the skin and production of airborne particles. Unfortunately, the term *latex* may also be used to describe a suspension of particles, and not these natural rubber latex products. This is the case with latex paint, which does not contain natural rubber latex and need not be avoided by latex-allergic individuals.

Epidemiology

Despite the prevalance of latex sensitivity (as defined by the presence of latex-specific IgE) in 9–37% of the general population [3], the **prevalence of clinical LA** is <1% [1]. Estimates of sensitization among health care workers are variable, most ranging between 5 and 17%. However, there is a lack of definite evidence demonstrating an increased risk of sensitization or immediate hypersensitivity to latex in this group [4]. The increased prevalence of LA among patients with spina bifida (50%) is highly reported; however, it is not limited to children with this disease. Sensitivity to natural rubber latex has been found in 34.1% of children with a history of three or more surgical interventions [5]. Although there was a dramatic increase in reported LA with the institution of universal precautions in the 1980s, recent years have seen a decrease in the incidence of LA, likely secondary to improvements in the manufacturing process and better definition of the disease. Anaphylaxis to latex does occur, but is rare, with an estimated incidence of 220 cases/yr in the United States [6].

CAUSES

Pathogenesis

Approximately **15 potential latex allergens** have been identified using molecular techniques [1]. Hev b 1 and Hev b 3 are major allergens for children with multiple congenital anomalies, whereas Hev b 2 and Hev b 4 are involved in LA among health care workers. Hev b 5 plays a major role in both groups [1]. Immunologic and/or clinical **cross-reactivity with foods,** including chestnut, avocado, kiwi, banana, tomato, and potato, has been detected [1]. Latex-allergic individuals should avoid these foods.

PRESENTATION

Risk Factors

The principal risk factor in sensitization to latex allergens is exposure. This increased exposure is thought to be responsible for the higher prevalence of LA in at-risk groups such as children with spina bifida and children who have undergone multiple surgeries. Atopy is noted to be a risk factor in adults with LA but not necessarily in children with spina bifida. Given this information, and the sensitivity of health care workers to different latex allergens, it is possible that adults represent a different population of latex allergic individuals than the spina bifida population. However, the clinical differences between these groups have not yet been well studied. Individuals with allergy to the foods listed above are also thought to be at increased risk of LA. Specific risk factors for anaphylaxis to latex are not known.

Exposure may occur by cutaneous, percutaneous, mucosal, or parenteral routes. Direct mucosal and parenteral exposure routes are associated with the greatest risk for anaphylaxis. Patients with previously limited cutaneous or respiratory irritation may have a more severe reaction when exposed through the mucosal or parenteral route.

Clinical Presentation

Contact reactions to latex gloves include the following:

- **IgE-mediated hypersensitivity** in the form of contact urticaria is the most common presentation of true LA [7]. It occurs within minutes of contact. With progressive sensitization, generalized urticaria, angioedema, rhinoconjunctivitis, bronchospasm, or anaphylaxis can occur on contact exposure.
- **Contact dermatitis** is not technically allergic in nature but may be described by some patients as LA and occurs with much higher frequency than true LA. Erythema, pruritus, and vesicles with crusting may appear 24–48 hrs after contact, mostly on the dorsum of the hands. It occurs through a type IV hypersensitivity, primarily to mercaptobenzothiazole and tetramethyl thiuram accelerators added in the manufacturing process [6].
- **Irritant contact dermatitis** does not have an immunologic basis. It presents with erythema, infiltration, scaling, and fissures on the dorsum of the hand and is usually due to occlusion, mechanical irritation, alkaline glove pH, or sweat.

Inhalant exposure to latex allergens adsorbed by cornstarch powder may also induce symptoms representative of type I immediate hypersensitivity, including nasal and ocular symptoms, urticaria, wheezing, and anaphylactic shock.

Anaphylaxis occurs most commonly with mucosal exposure but can occur with contact or inhalational exposure.

DIAGNOSIS

Any diagnostic test demonstrating latex-specific IgE must be interpreted in the context of the clinical history.

Serologic tests for the detection of latex-specific IgE include the CAP System FEIA (Pharmacia), Microplate AlaSTAT (Diagnostic Products Corporation), and HY-TEC EIA (HYCOR Biomedical, Inc.). In a comparative study, the Pharmacia CAP and DPC AlaSTAT assays produced 25% false-negative results, whereas the HY-TEC assay produced 27% false-positive results [1]. Thus, a negative result by the Pharmacia CAP or DPC AlaSTAT assay or a positive result by HY-TEC assay must be interpreted in the context of the clinical suspicion for LA.

Standardized extract for skin prick testing is not yet available in the United States. Some institutions may perform skin testing using extract made in their own labs from purchased latex gloves. As with any type of skin testing, it should be carried out only in the presence of trained personnel and resuscitation equipment.

Patch testing using a standard screening panel containing 1% p-phenylenediamine, 1% mercaptobenzothiazole, 1% mercapto mix, 1% thiuram mix, and 3% carba mix may help distinguish irritant dermatitis from contact dermatitis caused by a delayed hypersensitivity mechanism [6]. Small pieces of latex glove are sometimes used for patch testing, but this testing is less standardized than the screening panel and may be more difficult to interpret.

A **provocational challenge study** may be considered in a patient with a clinical history that strongly supports LA without confirmation from serologic or skin prick testing:

- **In glove-use tests,** the patient wears a latex glove for 15–60 mins while observed for the development of contact or inhalational symptoms. Patient blinding is difficult, and the variable latex content of gloves introduces the risk of systemic allergic reaction.
- **The Modified Glove Provocational Protocol** involves puncture of the skin followed by application of a high-allergen-content latex glove. The patient wears goggles and a respirator while being observed for symptoms.
- **The Hooded Exposure Chamber** allows graded latex aeroallergen exposure to the conjunctiva, upper airway, and lower airway using latex-associated cornstarch particles. This method allows quantitation of allergen exposure and result data, allows patient blinding, and is safer and more sensitive than other challenge methods, although it is time consuming and labor intensive [7].

MANAGEMENT

Management of LA focuses on prevention and avoidance.

Screening questions should be asked of patients on hospital admission and before planned surgical procedures to identify patients with possible latex sensitization (Table 17-1). Once LA is detected, the patient should wear a medical alert bracelet or necklace and carry an epinephrine injection pen at all times.

Complete **latex avoidance** may be unachievable and unnecessary other than for those with a history of a life-threatening reaction [1]. At the minimum, all latex gloves and products should be removed from the vicinity of the patient. "Hypoallergenic" latex gloves or powder-free latex gloves are not safe substitutes and should not be present in the room of any patient with LA. Resuscitation equipment should be available at all times. Surgical procedures should take place in a latex-free OR. *In vitro* studies reveal that washing powdered gloves does not have an effect on the amount of antigen transfer [6].

Alternatives to latex gloves include vinyl, nitrile, neoprene, and styrene gloves. Vinyl gloves are similar in cost to latex gloves but are less protective against viral penetration. Neoprene and styrene gloves are used mostly for surgical purposes and are five to ten times more expensive than latex gloves [8]. In simulated-use testing, nitrile gloves appear most comparable to latex gloves [1]. However, they are produced with mercaptobenzothiazole, the same accelerator used in the production of latex gloves, and thus they may still cause irritant or contact dermatitis reactions [8].

TABLE 17-1. SCREENING QUESTIONS FOR IDENTIFICATION OF LATEX SENSITIVITY

Have you had any past skin reaction, nasal or ocular allergic reaction, difficulty breathing, cough or wheezing, or anaphylactic shock reaction after contact with gloves, condoms, balloons, or other latex-containing products, or after a medical or dental procedure?

Do you have a personal or family history of atopy (allergies, hives, eczema, or asthma)?

Do you have a history of multiple surgeries or catheterizations?

Have you had any past allergic reaction to avocado, banana, chestnut, kiwi, potato, or tomato?

TABLE 17-2. MEDICAL AND HOUSEHOLD PRODUCTS THAT MAY CONTAIN LATEX

Medical	Household
Gloves	Toys
Catheters (including urinary catheters and wound drains)	Balloons
	Elastic on clothing
Tape	Mouse pads
Electrode pads	Condoms
Rubber syringe stoppers	Shoes
Tourniquets	Erasers
Face masks	Sporting goods
Ambu bags	Rubber handles on tools
Mattresses	Buttons on stereos, video cassette recorders, televisions, and remote controls
Patient-controlled analgesia syringes	
Stethoscope and BP cuff tubing	

The FDA has established guidelines for labeling of any medical devices containing latex. A brief list of medical and household products that may contain latex, as well as resources for the identification of latex products and latex-free substitutes for the medical and home environments, is given in Table 17-2.

Further information, including lists of latex products and latex-free substitutes, is available from the Spina Bifida Association of America (800-621-3141 or http://www.sbaa.org) and the American Latex Allergy Association (888-97-ALERT or http://www.latexallergyresources.org).

KEY POINTS

- LA is an immediate hypersensitivity reaction caused by exposure to natural rubber latex.
- Any diagnostic test demonstrating latex-specific IgE must be interpreted in the context of clinical history.
- Management of LA focuses on avoidance of exposure to latex. Screening questions (such as a history of past reactions to latex or cross-reactive foods) should be asked of patients before planned surgical procedures to identify patients with possible latex sensitization.

REFERENCES

1. Poley, Jr GE, Slater JE. Latex allergy. *J Allergy Clin Immunol* 2000;105:1054–1062.
2. Woods JA, Lambert S, Platts-Mills TAE, et al. Natural rubber latex allergy: spectrum, diagnostic approach, and therapy. *J Emerg Med* 1997;15:71–85.
3. Garabrant DH, Roth HD, Parsad R, et al. Latex sensitization in health care workers and in the US general population. *Am J Epidemiol* 2001;153:515–522.
4. Garabrant DH, Schweitzer S. Epidemiology of latex sensitization and allergies in health care workers. *J Allergy Clin Immunol* 2002;110:582–595.
5. Brehler R, Kütting B. Natural rubber latex allergy: a problem of interdisciplinary concern in medicine. *Arch Intern Med* 2001;161:1057–1064.
6. Neuget AI, Ghatak AT, Miller RL. Anaphylaxis in the United States: an investigation into its epidemiology. *Arch Intern Med* 2001;161:15–21.
7. Kurtz KM, Hamilton RG, Adkinson NF. Role and application of provocation in the diagnosis of occupational latex allergy. *Ann Allergy Asthma Immunol* 1999; 83:634–639.
8. Reddy S. Latex allergy. *Am Fam Physician* 1998;57:93–100.

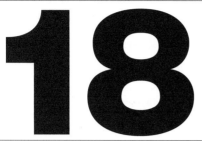

Conditions Associated with Eosinophilia

Barbara C. Jost

INTRODUCTION

Eosinophilia is seen in association with a broad spectrum of disorders ranging from allergic to malignant diseases.

Definition

Eosinophilia is defined by an absolute eosinophil count $\geq 0.7 \times 10^9$/L. However, the upper limit of normal in most laboratories is 0.35×10^9/L.

Classification

The patient with eosinophilia may be classified into one of five categories, depending on the clinical context (e.g., malignancy or infection) or the organ system that dominates the clinical picture (Table 18-1).

Incidental Eosinophilia
Incidental eosinophilia discovered on a routine blood count may arise from

- **Infection**, most likely parasitic.
- **Drugs.** Drug-related eosinophilia may be associated with one or more of the following: cutaneous lesions (beta-lactams), hepatitis (phenothiazines, methotrexate, allopurinol), hypersensitivity vasculitis (phenytoin), or pulmonary infiltrates (see Drug Reactions).
  Eosinophilia-myalgia syndrome is a rare drug-related eosinophilia that was epidemic in the late 1980s. It was ultimately linked to a contaminant in L-tryptophan preparations that were recalled by the FDA in 1990. In addition to peripheral eosinophilia and myalgias, pulmonary involvement was noted in 50–60% of cases.
- **Asthma**
- **Collagen vascular disease** (e.g., Churg-Strauss vasculitis, rheumatoid arthritis, eosinophilic fasciitis)
- **Inflammatory bowel disease**
- **Malignancy**
- **Idiopathic hypereosinophilic syndrome (HES).** This should be considered in any patient who has a persistent elevation in total eosinophil count of $>1.5 \times 10^9$/L for >6 mos and in whom there is no evidence for commonly recognized causes of eosinophilia (Table 18-2) despite careful evaluation. HES is also characterized by multiorgan damage due to extensive infiltrates of mature eosinophils. Examples of end-organ damage in HES include restrictive cardiomyopathy; endocardial fibrosis; peripheral neuropathy; polymyositis; arteritis affecting GI tract, lung, kidney, and skin; and pulmonary infiltrates or pleural effusions. 40% of patients with HES have evidence of pulmonary involvement. HES is also associated with a hypercoagulable state that contributes to the development of thromboembolic disease. More than half of patients have constitutional symptoms such as fever, weight loss, and night sweats. Prognosis is poor, with a mean survival of just 9 mos without treatment (see Treatment).

TABLE 18-1. CLASSIFICATION SCHEME FOR EOSINOPHILIA

Incidental eosinophilia
Pulmonary infiltrates with eosinophilia
Cutaneous lesions with eosinophilia
Parasitic infection with eosinophilia
Malignancy with eosinophilia

Pulmonary Infiltrates with Eosinophilia (PIE Syndromes)

Löffler first described the syndrome of pulmonary infiltrates with peripheral eosinophilia in 1932 (Löffler's syndrome) [1]. The PIE syndromes may be divided into two groups, depending on the presence or absence of asthma (Table 18-3).

- **Chronic eosinophilic pneumonia** is characterized by the insidious onset (i.e., >1 mo) of cough, fever and sweats, dyspnea, and weight loss. The female to male ratio is 2:1. Peak incidence is in the fifth decade. An estimated 33–40% of patients have asthma. Thus, this disease can occur either in the presence or absence of asthma. Radiographic findings and diagnostic considerations are described in Table 18-4. Early treatment with corticosteroids is usually rapidly effective, but the disease often recurs and may become refractory to corticosteroid treatment.
- **Churg-Strauss syndrome (CSS)** is characterized by hypereosinophilia and systemic vasculitis in patients with underlying asthma. The typical presentation is a patient with known asthma who exhibits sinus disease, neuropathy (mono- or poly-), and systemic symptoms such as fever, weight loss, and fatigue. Multiple other organs may be affected with vasculitis, including the skin, heart, kidney, or CNS. Asthma and eosinophilia precede the systemic vasculitis in 40% of patients. At this stage, the patient is considered to have *formes frustes* of CSS. Diagnostic criteria are summarized in Table 18-4. A serum ANCA test is a useful screening test for CSS, but a negative test result does not rule out the diagnosis. Roughly 40–60% of

TABLE 18-2. CONDITIONS ASSOCIATED WITH PERIPHERAL EOSINOPHILIA

Most common	Less common
Asthma	Eosinophilia-myalgia syndrome
Drug-related	Eosinophilic fasciitis (Schulman's syndrome)
Parasitic infection	
Idiopathic hypereosinophilic syndrome	Metastatic colon, lung, breast, cervical, ovarian carcinomas
Pulmonary infiltrate with eosinophilia syndromes	Psoriasis
	Rheumatoid arthritis
Churg-Strauss syndrome	Other collagen vascular diseases
Atopic dermatitis	Inflammatory bowel disease
Bullous pemphigoid	Myelodysplastic syndrome
	Myeloproliferative disorders
	Plasma cell dyscrasias
	Lymphoma
	Leukemia

TABLE 18-3. CLASSIFICATION OF PULMONARY INFILTRATES WITH EOSINOPHILIA (PIE) SYNDROMES

PIE with asthma	PIE without asthma
Chronic eosinophilic pneumonia	Infection and infestation (Löffler's syndrome)
Churg-Strauss syndrome (allergic granulomatosis)	Chronic eosinophilic pneumonia
	Drug reaction
Allergic bronchopulmonary aspergillosis	Pulmonary eosinophilic granuloma
	Bronchocentric granulomatosis
Tropical eosinophilia	Neoplasia
	Idiopathic hypereosinophilic syndrome

Modified from Karr RM, Salvaggio JE. Infiltrative hypersensitivity disease of the lung. In: Parker CW, ed. *Clinical immunology*. Philadelphia: WB Saunders, 1980; 1336–1371.

cases of CSS will have a positive test (usually p-ANCA). Treatment is with high-dose corticosteroids. Cyclophosphamide is reserved for slow responders or patients who relapse during steroid taper.
- **Allergic bronchopulmonary aspergillosis** is discussed in Chap. 4, Asthma.
- **Tropical eosinophilia (or parasitic infection).** In the United States, *Strongyloides* (strongyloidiasis), *Ascaris* (ascariasis), *Toxocara* (visceral larva migrans), and *Ancylostoma* (hookworm disease) are the most common parasites causing pulmonary infiltrates. Other helminthic parasitic infections seen in the United States include trichinosis (*Trichinella*) and hookworm disease caused by *Necator*. Tropical eosinophilia is caused by filarial worms such as *Wuchereria bancrofti* and *Brugia malayi*. The male to female ratio is 4:1; peak incidence is in the third or fourth decade. Constitutional symptoms (fever, weight loss, fatigue), nocturnal productive cough and wheezing, hemoptysis, and dyspnea are insidious in onset. Treatment is with anti-helminthics.
- **Löffler's syndrome (simple pulmonary eosinophilia)** is characterized by minimal or no symptoms in the setting of migratory infiltrates on chest x-ray and eosinophilia. The syndrome is thought to represent a hypersensitivity response to a number of causative agents, including a variety of drugs (including sulfonamides, chlorpropamide, nitrofurantoin), chemicals (including nickel), and parasites. Many patients are ultimately diagnosed as having a drug reaction or parasitic infection. The disease typically resolves spontaneously within 1 mo.
- **Acute eosinophilic pneumonia (AEP)** is characterized by the acute onset (over 1–5 days) of fever, pleuritic chest pain, hypoxemic respiratory failure, and myalgias in the setting of diffuse pulmonary infiltrates and eosinophilia both peripherally and in bronchoalveolar lavage fluid. The cause remains unknown. It has been proposed that AEP represents an acute hypersensitivity phenomenon [2]—e.g., to inhaled allergens such as *Trichosporon*. Associations with drugs (e.g., NSAIDs, antidepressants), smoking (particularly initiation of smoking), and parasitic infection have been reported. There is typically a dramatic response to steroids.
- **Drug reaction** (see also Hypersensitivity Syndrome). More than 30 drugs have been reported to cause eosinophilia and pulmonary infiltrates (e.g., methotrexate, nitrofurantoin, sulfa compounds, gold, salicylates, antiepileptics). Presentation can vary from mild (e.g., simple pulmonary eosinophilia) to severe (e.g., acute eosinophilic pneumonia). Likewise, treatment varies from simple cessation of the medication to corticosteroids.
- **Pulmonary eosinophilic granuloma (PEG)** is a rare, fibroinflammatory disorder characterized by a mixed interstitial infiltrate of eosinophils, lymphocytes, and Langerhans' cells. PEG is a subtype of the Langerhans' cell histiocytoses, formerly

TABLE 18-4. DIAGNOSTIC FEATURES OF SELECTED PULMONARY INFILTRATES WITH EOSINOPHILIA (PIE) SYNDROMES

PIE syndrome	Radiographic features	Diagnosis
Löffler's syndrome	Migrating, transient nonsegmental infiltrates	Minimally symptomatic + history of exposure to parasites/drugs + spontaneous resolution
Chronic eosinophilic pneumonia	"Photographic negative of pulmonary edema" [4] and subpleural consolidation	Insidious clinical course (cough, anorexia, weight loss) + typical chest x-ray + response to steroids
Acute eosinophilic pneumonia	Diffuse bilateral reticular densities	Acute clinical course + response to steroids
Churg-Strauss syndrome	Transient, patchy, nonsegmental consolidation	At least 4 out of the following 6 criteria: asthma, eosinophilia >10%, mono- or polyneuropathy, pulmonary infiltrates, sinus abnormalities, extravascular extension of eosinophils on lung biopsy
ABPA	Pulmonary infiltrates, central bronchiectasis, "finger-in-glove" sign (medium-sized bronchi with mucus)	Asthma, eosinophilia, (+)-skin test to *Aspergillus fumigatus*, (+)-serum precipitins, markedly elevated serum IgE levels, typical chest x-ray
Parasitic infection	Fine diffuse reticulonodular lesions preferentially in lower lung zones	Exposure history, stool exam for ova and parasites or parasitic antigens, serologies
Drug reaction	Consolidation, hilar adenopathy, pleural effusion or reticulonodular densities [5]	Clinical correlation, response to drug withdrawal
Bronchocentric granulomatosis	Focal mass or lobar consolidation with atelectasis [6]	Biopsy
Hypereosinophilic syndrome	Patchy reticular densities, poorly defined nodules, and consolidation; cardiomegaly, pleural effusion	>1.5 × 10^9/L eosinophils for ≥ 6 mos, multi-organ dysfunction

referred to as the *histiocytosis X disorders* (Letterer-Siwe syndrome, Hand-Schüller-Christian disease, and eosinophilic granuloma). In eosinophilic granuloma, the medullary cavity of any bone in the skeletal system may be primarily affected by an erosive and expanding accumulation of cells. PEG is characterized by the insidious onset of cough in the setting of these bony lesions. There is evidence that PEG is associated with smoking, and, indeed, remissions have been documented after cessation of smoking. Spontaneous pneumothorax is linked to PEG. PEG may regress spontaneously or progress to fibrotic lung disease.

- **Bronchocentric granulomatosis** is characterized by mild symptoms, including fever, cough, chest pain, and hemoptysis. Approximately two-thirds of cases occur in nonasthmatics. Mean age of onset is 50 for nonasthmatics and 20 for asthmatics. Mycobacterial or fungal infections have been associated with bronchocentric granulomatosis in nonasthmatics.
- **Neoplasias.** Lymphoma is the most common neoplasia associated with pulmonary infiltrates and eosinophilia. Chronic eosinophilic pneumonia has been described in cutaneous T cell lymphoma [3]. Acute lymphoblastic leukemia has also been associated with PIE syndromes.
- **Idiopathic hypereosinophilic syndrome** (HES).

Cutaneous Lesions with Eosinophilia

- **Drug-related eosinophilia** may be associated with cutaneous lesions in the case of the beta-lactams.
- **Hypersensitivity syndrome (HSS)** refers to a severe idiosyncratic cutaneous adverse drug reaction associated with multiorgan involvement (e.g., hepatitis, myocarditis, interstitial pneumonitis, interstitial nephritis, and thyroiditis), blood eosinophilia (typically $>1.5 \times 10^9$/L), and sometimes lymphocytosis. Lymphadenopathy and high-grade fever are common findings. Onset is delayed, typically 2–8 wks after initiation of therapy. Skin lesions are diffusely distributed, slowly evolving, and pruritic in nature [7]. The most common offenders are the aromatic antiepileptic agents (phenytoin, carbamazepine, and phenobarbital), with an estimated incidence of one reaction/5,000 patients (higher among black patients). Other offenders include the sulfonamides. HSS has also been reported with dapsone, allopurinol, and minocycline.
- **Atopic dermatitis** (see Chap. 10, Atopic Dermatitis).
- **Bullous pemphigoid** is a vesiculobullous disease that can be localized or generalized and can be limited to the skin or involve mucosal surfaces. It often provokes blood and tissue eosinophilia.
- **Psoriasis** is a common chronic inflammatory dermatosis that may be associated with eosinophilia.

Parasitic Infection with Eosinophilia

The most common parasitic infections associated with eosinophilia in North America are visceral larva migrans (*Toxocara*), ascariasis (*Ascaris*), trichinosis (*Trichinella*), hookworm disease (*Ancylostoma* and *Necator*), and strongyloidiasis (*Strongyloides*).

Malignancy with Eosinophilia

The most common malignancies associated with peripheral eosinophilia are lymphoma (particularly Hodgkin's disease), metastatic solid tumor disease, and myelodysplastic syndrome. The presence of peripheral eosinophilia in the setting of malignancy is a marker of extensive disease and poor prognosis.

CAUSES

Pathophysiology

Eosinophils are bone marrow–derived granulocytes involved in allergic and non-allergic inflammation. They survive for only 6–12 hrs in the circulation, but after passing into tissue, they may survive for weeks. Eosinophils store and release large quantities of **preformed cytotoxic basic proteins** from cytoplasmic granules. These include eosinophil major basic protein, eosinophil cationic protein, eosinophil peroxidase, and eosinophil-derived neurotoxin. Eosinophils also produce superoxide, leukotrienes, and cytokines. Cytotoxic basic proteins released by eosinophils are involved in the host defense against parasites, but when deposited adjacent to host cells, these proteins can cause considerable damage by promoting inflammation, thrombosis, angiogenesis, and connective tissue formation. Eosinophilia is induced by eosinophil-stimulating cytokines, including interleukin-5, GM-CSF, and interleukin-3. These same cytokines are responsible for eosinophilopoiesis and prolongation of eosinophil survival in tissues. The latter process is due to inhibition of eosinophil apoptosis. There is an important diurnal variation of blood eosinophil levels, with highest counts occurring at night. Eosinophil counts also vary with age and activity. The presence of increased numbers of eosinophils in tissue generally indicates a pathologic condition. In certain diseases, such as eosinophilia-myalgia syndrome, extracellular deposition of eosinophil basic proteins, such as major basic protein, may be present long after tissue eosinophils are no longer detected.

Differential Diagnosis

Allergic diseases are the most common cause of eosinophilia in North America, whereas parasitic infection is the most common cause worldwide.

Conditions associated with peripheral eosinophilia are listed in Table 18-2.

The **degree of eosinophilia** may serve as an important clue to the underlying cause.

- **Mild eosinophilia**, $<1.5 \times 10^9/L$, is most often due to allergic states or drug reactions.
- **Marked eosinophilia**, usually defined as $>5 \times 10^9/L$, is seen during the tissue migration phase of parasitic infection (i.e., larval stage) and in the hypereosinophilic syndrome.
- **Moderate eosinophilia** is occasionally seen in allergic states but raises the possibility of a more serious underlying condition (see Table 18-2).

PRESENTATION

Evaluation

Eosinophilia may be discovered on a routine blood count (incidental finding) or as a result of a high degree of clinical suspicion based on a careful history. An approach to evaluation of the patient with eosinophilia follows.

History

A careful **medication history** may uncover a temporal relationship between eosinophilia and starting a new medication. It is important to recognize that *the overall incidence of eosinophilia in all patients taking medication is very low*.

A detailed **travel history** is necessary, as travel to tropical regions, such as Africa or Asia, may point to parasitic infestation as a possible cause of eosinophilia. The temporal relationship of symptom onset to travel should be ascertained.

The **social history** should focus on possible home or occupational exposure to allergens.

Review of systems is particularly helpful in the evaluation of eosinophilia. Patients should be thoroughly questioned about allergic symptoms such as dry, itchy, scaly skin (atopic dermatitis) and wheezing, chest tightness, and shortness of breath (asthma). Symptoms referable to collagen vascular disease (e.g., rash, joint pain, fever, xerostomia), inflammatory bowel disease (e.g., diarrhea, abdominal pain, joint pain, skin lesions), malignancy (e.g., weight loss, night sweats, lymphadenopathy), and parasitic infection (e.g., diarrhea, weight loss, rash) should also be elicited.

Clinical Evaluation

Clinical evaluation should include basic lab work, such as a comprehensive metabolic panel (electrolytes, liver function tests, creatinine, calcium, total protein) and a chest x-ray. **Absolute eosinophil counts**, rather than percentages of the total white cell count attributable to eosinophils, should be used to monitor eosinophilia. If a vasculitic syndrome is suspected, an ANCA test should be performed.

In the event of a suspected drug reaction, **cessation of the suspect drug** is the first step.

In the presence of respiratory symptoms not attributable to asthma, a **chest x-ray** may reveal evidence of one of the PIE syndromes. Radiographic findings and diagnostic considerations for the PIE syndromes are outlined in Table 18-4.

If symptoms of allergic rhinitis or asthma are present, **limited skin testing** for common aeroallergens should be considered.

If parasitic infection is in the differential diagnosis, **exam of the stool for ova and parasites** or parasitic antigens should be completed. Serologic testing for endemic parasites is also indicated.

If a cause of eosinophilia is not found, a CBC should be repeated in 1–2 mos. If eosinophilia $>1.5 \times 10^9$/L persists for >6 mos without an obvious cause, then the patient meets criteria for HES (see Idiopathic Hypereosinophilia Syndrome).

MANAGEMENT

Treatment

Treatment of eosinophilia is predicated on **treatment of the underlying condition**—e.g., antihelminthics for parasitic infections, chemotherapeutics for underlying malignancy. Corticosteroids are used for many of the PIE syndromes (see Pulmonary Infiltrates with Eosinophilia), including ABPA, chronic eosinophilic pneumonia, and CSS. Cytoxan is recommended in CSS that is refractory to corticosteroids. For treatment of HES, cytotoxic agents, such as hydroxyurea, vincristine, 6-mercaptopurine, and cyclosporine, have been shown to improve survival [8]. Newer studies have focused on interferon-alpha alone or in combination with hydroxyurea for the treatment of HES [9]. A humanized anti-IL5 antibody is being studied in patients with HES. Stem cell transplantation is also under investigation.

KEY POINTS

- Allergic diseases are the most common cause of eosinophilia in North America; parasitic infection is the most common cause worldwide.
- The absolute eosinophil count, not percentage of eosinophils, should be used to monitor eosinophilia.
- Treatment of eosinophilia is predicated on treatment of the underlying condition.

REFERENCES

1. Löffler W. Zur differential-diagnose der lungeninfiltrierungen. Il uber fluchtige succedan-infiltrate (mit eosinophilie). *Beitr Klin Tuberk* 1932;79:368–392.
2. Badesch DB, King TE Jr, Schwartz MI. Acute eosinophilic pneumonia: a hypersensitivity phenomenon? *Am Rev Respir Dis* 1989;139:249–252.
3. Hirshberg B, Kramer MR, Lotem M, et al. Chronic eosinophilic pneumonia associated with cutaneous T-cell lymphoma. *Am J Hematol* 1999;60(2):143–147.
4. Gaensler EA, Carrington CB. Peripheral opacities in chronic eosinophilic pneumonia: the photographic negative of pulmonary edema. *AJR Am J Roentgenol* 1977;128:1–13.
5. Kim Y, Lee KS, Choi DC, et al. The spectrum of eosinophilic lung disease: radiologic findings. *J Comput Assist Tomogr* 1997;21(6):920–930.
6. Ward S, Heyneman LE, Flint JD, et al. Bronchocentric granulomatosis: computed tomographic findings in five patients. *Clin Radiol* 2000;55(4):296–300.
7. Roujeau J-C, Stern RS. Severe adverse cutaneous reactions to drugs. *N Engl J Med* 1994;331:1272–1285.
8. Liesveld JL, Abboud CN. Leukocyte disorders. State of the art: the hypereosinophilic syndromes. *Blood Rev* 1991;529–537.
9. Malbrain MLNG, van den Bergh H, Zachee P. Further evidence for the clonal nature of the idiopathic hypereosinophilic syndrome: complete haematological and cytogenetic remission induced by interferon-alpha in a case with a unique chromosomal abnormality. *Br J Haematol* 1996;92:176–183.

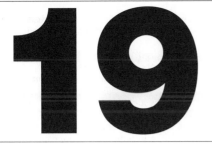

Mastocytosis

Elizabeth C. Friedman

INTRODUCTION

Definition

The mast cell is one of the main effectors of the allergic response. Mastocytosis is an abnormal proliferation of mast cells. Although the disease is rare, it can occur at any age. Features of the disease include pruritus, urtication, flushing, nausea, vomiting, diarrhea, abdominal pain, vascular instability, headache, and neuropsychiatric problems. The disease has been classified into four categories, some of which are associated with hematologic disorders and malignancies. In general, treatment is supportive.

Classification

I. Indolent mastocytosis
    A. Cutaneous
        1. Urticaria pigmentosa
        2. Diffuse cutaneous mastocytosis
        3. Mastocytoma
        4. Telangiectasia macularis eruptiva perstans
    B. Systemic
II. Mastocytosis with associated hematologic disorder
III. Aggressive mastocytosis
IV. Mastocytic leukemia

CAUSES

Pathogenesis

Mast cells display a vast array of antigens on their cell surface, as do all cells of the immune system. These surface antigens regulate activation or cell recognition or act as cytokine receptors. They are abnormal or disregulated in various inflammatory states and diseases, including mastocytosis. It has recently been reported that mast cells from patients with mastocytosis and mast cell leukemia display surface antigens, which normal mast cells do not. Previously, it was widely speculated that the protooncogene c-kit and its ligand stem cell factor play a role in mast cell disease.

PRESENTATION

Typical Skin Findings

90% of pediatric and adult patients with indolent mastocytosis have **urticaria pigmentosa** (UP). They consist of yellowish-tan to reddish-brown macular-papular lesions. The palms, soles, face, and scalp are usually spared. UP lesions respond to mechanical stroking with urtication (raised wheal and erythema), referred to as *Darier's sign*.

Diffuse cutaneous mastocytosis is seen in children >3 yrs old. Usually all skin is involved and has a normal to yellow-brown appearance. It is often thickened.

Bullous eruptions with hemorrhage are generally seen in children with either UP or diffuse cutaneous mastocytosis.

Mastocytomas are solitary lesions consisting of nests of mast cells. These are fairly rare, appear before 6 mos of age, and involute over time.

Telangiectasia eruptiva macularis perstans is a very rare presentation of mastocytosis affecting <1% of adults with the disease. The lesions are subtle, consisting of patchy erythema and macules of variable coloration ranging from tan to brown with overlying telangiectasia.

Systemic Symptoms

Systemic symptoms depend on which organ system is involved and **can be seen in the absence of cutaneous lesions**. Mastocytosis should be in a differential diagnosis for flushing syndromes (e.g., carcinoid and pheochromocytoma), especially when accompanied by hypotension.

- **Bone marrow**: The most common extracutaneous site of involvement. On a trephine core biopsy, mast cells resemble fibroblasts and histiocytes. They can only be distinguished by specific stains. Infiltration by mast cells can have osteolytic activity; thus, a bone scan is necessary once diagnosed in the marrow.
- **GI**: Diarrhea, nausea, and vomiting are presumably from mast cell degranulation within the GI tract.
- **Liver**: Elevated alkaline phosphatase and gamma-glutamyltransferase are seen secondary to mast cell invasion. Rarely causes serious disease.
- **Spleen**: Trabecular, fibrotic thickening is most commonly seen.

MANAGEMENT

Workup

- History
- Physical exam
- Skin biopsy
- Bone marrow biopsy
- 24-hour urine for 5-hydroxyindoleacetic acid; urinary metanephrines to rule out carcinoid and pheochromocytoma

Treatment

The goal of therapy is control of mast cell mediators, primarily histamine.

- Antihistamines: hydroxyzine (Atarax), cetirizine (Zyrtec) (less sedating), often in large doses to control pruritus. Doxepin (Sinequan) (a tricyclic antidepressant), although very sedating, is also very good at controlling pruritus.
- Cromolyn sodium (Gastrochrom): mast cell stabilizer. Can be very helpful when taken orally for GI symptoms.
- Epinephrine (EpiPen, EpiPen Jr.) for anaphylaxis. Patients should be taught how to use it and carry it with them.
- PUVA for extensive skin involvement.
- Topical steroids: use with caution, because although they may induce a remission of UP lesions for up to a year, lesions generally recur, and the patient would be at risk for skin atrophy from repeated use.

- H_2-blockers for GI symptoms. Anticholinergics can be helpful for diarrhea, although this symptom is often difficult to treat.
- Oral steroids: Use with caution to avoid side effects. Can be helpful for GI symptoms.

Prognosis

- 50% of children with isolated UP will resolve by adulthood.
- Adults with UP tend to develop systemic involvement.
- Category I often progresses to II.
- Patients with hematologic disease generally have a poor prognosis. Mast cell leukemia has a mean survival of 6 mos.

KEY POINTS

- Systemic mastocytosis can occur in the absence of cutaneous syndromes.
- Mastocytosis should be part of any workup for flushing syndromes.

SUGGESTED READING

Chines A, Korenblat PE, et al. Systemic mastocytosis presenting as osteoporosis: a clinical and histomorphometric study. *J Clin Endocrinol Metab* 1991;72:141–144.

Worobec AS, Metcalfe DD. Mastocytosis: current treatment concepts. *Int Arch Allergy Immunol* 2002;127:153–155.

Metcalfe DD. Mastocytosis syndromes. In: Middleton E, Reed CE, Ellis EF, eds. *Allergy, principles and practice*, 5th ed. St. Louis: Mosby, 1998.

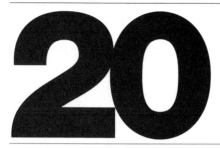

Primary Immunodeficiency Diseases

Barbara C. Jost

INTRODUCTION

Primary immunodeficiency diseases (PIDs) are a diverse group of diseases characterized by immune system dysfunction causing **increased susceptibility to infection** and **abnormal inflammatory responses**. PID is generally considered a topic largely within the realm of pediatrics. This chapter focuses on the aspects of PID most relevant to the internist. Practitioners focusing on the care of the adult patient may be faced with general health management of patients with PID diagnosed during childhood, or they may be considering the diagnosis of PID in a patient with recurrent infection. The former scenario requires at least a working knowledge of the classification and manifestations of PID, whereas the latter scenario requires familiarity with a basic diagnostic scheme.

Epidemiology

PID is rare. There are >70 distinct PIDs recognized by the World Health Organization (WHO) Scientific Group on PID, affecting an estimated 500,000 individuals in the United States [1]. The most common PID is IgA deficiency, affecting one in 700 individuals, though it is often clinically inapparent. Common variable immunodeficiency affects an estimated 7,000 individuals in the United States. The prevalence of chronic granulomatous disease, estimated by a U.S. registry established in 1992, is at least four per million [2]. Most cases of PID are diagnosed in infancy or early childhood.

Classification

The **classification scheme** adopted by the WHO Scientific Group on PID corresponds to the basic pathophysiology underlying this complex group of diseases.

- **Antibody, or B cell, deficiencies** comprise 50–60% of all PIDs.
- **Combined T and B cell deficiencies** comprise 20–25% of all PIDs.
- **T cell deficiencies** comprise 5–10% of all PIDs.
- **Complement deficiencies** comprise <2% of all PIDs.
- **Phagocytic cell, or granulocyte, disorders** comprise 10–15% of all PIDs.

A **genetic defect** has been identified for many PIDs. The majority are X-linked or autosomal recessive.

PRESENTATION

History

A history of recurrent, chronic, prolonged, complicated, severe, or opportunistic infections in a patient without known secondary immunodeficiency (e.g., malignancy, HIV/AIDS, immunosuppressive therapy, malnutrition) should prompt consideration of PID. Historical clues to the presence of PID are given in Table 20-1.

TABLE 20-1. HISTORICAL CLUES TO PRESENCE OF PRIMARY IMMUNODEFICIENCY DISEASES

Recurrent, chronic, or severe sinopulmonary (including otic) infections

Complicated sinopulmonary/otic infections

Recurrent or severe infections with encapsulated bacteria (e.g., pneumonia, meningitis, sepsis)

Need for repeated courses of antibiotics or treatment with gammaglobulin

Opportunistic infections

Wasting, failure to thrive

Recurrent or chronic diarrhea, malabsorption

Adverse reaction to live-virus immunization

Adverse reaction to blood or plasma transfusions (e.g., graft-versus-host disease in T cell deficiencies)

Recurrent infections of skin surface areas

Recurrent organ abscesses

Recurrent lymphadenitis

Recurrent periodontitis

Poor wound healing or post-surgical complications

Recurrent neisserial infections

Types and Patterns of Infection

- **Recurrent or chronic infections.** How many infections is too many? An often-cited guideline is >6–8 upper respiratory tract infections per year in the first decade of life or more than one episode of pneumonia per decade for adults. Also, any serious infection occurring twice in a child or once in an adult should raise suspicion of presence of a PID.
- **Prolonged duration** of infection.
- **Severe or complicated infections**, e.g., severe varicella complicated by pneumonia or hepatitis or bronchiectasis.
- **Infection with an opportunistic organism**, e.g., *Pneumocystis carinii* pneumonia (in absence of HIV).

Associated Features

The presence of other features or constellations of signs, such as cardiac disease, micrognathia, and hypocalcemia (DiGeorge syndrome); thrombocytopenia and eczema (Wiskott-Aldrich syndrome); and ataxia plus oculocutaneous telangiectasias (ataxia-telangiectasia syndrome), should prompt suspicion of PID.

Family History

Elements of the history that can also help aid in the diagnosis of PID are

- Family members with documented PID or recurrent infections
- Early infant deaths
- Autoimmune disease
- Consanguinity

Physical Exam

Clues to the presence of PID on exam and their associations are presented in Table 20-2.

**TABLE 20-2.   PHYSICAL EXAM FINDINGS IN PRIMARY
IMMUNODEFICIENCY DISEASE**

Exam finding	Association(s)
Failure to thrive	T cell deficiencies
Mucocutaneous candidiasis	Combined T and B cell deficiencies; Wiskott-Aldrich syndrome
Cutaneous ulcers, oral ulcers	Severe T cell deficiencies; hyper-IgM syndrome
Cutaneous abscesses	Phagocyte deficiencies; hyper-IgE syndrome
Atopic dermatitis	Wiskott-Aldrich syndrome; hyper-IgE syndrome; hypogammaglobulinemia
Telangiectasia	Ataxia-telangiectasia syndrome
Albinism (oculocutaneous)	Chediak-Higashi syndrome
Clubbing	Various
Recurrent otitis media, sinusitis	Various
Periodontitis	Phagocyte deficiencies
Small or absent tonsillar, adenoidal, peripheral lymph nodes	T cell deficiencies; B cell deficiencies
Lymphadenopathy, splenomegaly, hepatomegaly	Omenn syndrome; hyper-IgM syndrome; common variable immunodeficiency disease
Arthritis	Antibody deficiencies
Delayed umbilical cord detachment	Leukocyte adhesion defects

MANAGEMENT

Workup

Given the rarity of PID and the cost and potential morbidity associated with immunologic testing, a history compatible with PID is a prerequisite for embarking on a lab workup to confirm a clinical diagnosis of PID. Clinical presentation and the etiologic agents involved are the best clues to the class of PID suspected (Table 20-3). The lab evaluation is guided by the type of PID suspected [3] (Fig. 20-1 and Tables 20-4 through 20-7). A CBC and differential count should be ordered in all cases of suspected immunodeficiency.

Lab Evaluation for Suspected Antibody Deficiency
See Table 20-4 for a complete list.
   Rule out cystic fibrosis and immotile cilia syndrome (see Fig. 20-1). Cystic fibrosis presents with recurrent episodes of bronchitis, sinusitis, and pneumonia and is associated with malnutrition, failure to thrive, and steatorrhea. If features of the disease are present, **sweat chloride** should be used as a screening test (>60 mEq/L is abnormal in children; >80 mEq/L in adults). Sensitivity of this test is 80–85%. If the clinical suspicion is high, but the sweat test is negative or equivocal, genetic testing for cystic fibrosis transmembrane regulator gene mutations should be performed.
   Immotile cilia syndrome is characterized is an autosomal recessive condition characterized by immotility of the cilia of the sperm (infertility) and the airways (recurrent upper and lower respiratory infections, bronchiectasis).
   Quantitative immunoglobulins (IgG, IgM, IgA, IgE) should be interpreted according to age-related standards (refer to Appendix B). *Hypogammaglobulinemia* is

TABLE 20-3. COMMON PRESENTATIONS AND INFECTIOUS AGENTS CLASSIFIED BY PRIMARY IMMUNODEFICIENCY DISEASE SUBTYPE

Clinical presentation	Etiologic agents
Antibody deficiencies	
Sinusitis	*Streptococcus pneumoniae*
Pneumonia	*Haemophilus influenzae*
Pharyngitis	*Moraxella catarrhalis*
Otitis	*Neisseria meningitides*
Meningitis	*Staphylococcus aureus*
Bacteremia	*Pseudomonas*
Encephalitis (enteroviral)	Enterovirus (echovirus and poliovirus)
Colitis (giardiasis)	Rotavirus
	Giardia lamblia
	Cryptosporidium
	Mycoplasma (including *Ureaplasma urealyticum*)
Combined T and B cell deficiencies[a]	
Opportunistic infections	*Mycobacterium tuberculosis*
Failure to thrive	*Mycobacterium avium intracellulare*
Diarrhea	*Listeria monocytogenes*
Dermatitis	*Pneumocystis carinii*
Sepsis	*Toxoplasma*
	Cryptosporidium
	Cytomegalovirus
	Herpes simplex
	Herpes zoster
	Epstein-Barr virus
	Candida albicans
	Cryptococcus
	Nocardia
	Isospora belli
Phagocytic cell disorders	
Invasive skin infections/abscesses	*S. aureus*
Focal abscesses	*Pseudomonas cepacia*
Poor wound healing	*Salmonella typhimurium*
Lymphadenitis	*Serratia marcescens*
Periodontitis	*Escherichia coli*
	Mycobacterium fortuitum
	Aspergillus
	C. albicans
	Actinomyces
Complement deficiencies	
Pyogenic infections	*N. meningitides*[b]
	Neisseria gonorrheae[b]
	S. pneumoniae[c]

[a]May also see same clinical presentation and etiologic agents as are associated with antibody deficiency in combined T and B cell deficiency states.
[b]C5–C9 deficiency.
[c]C3 deficiency.

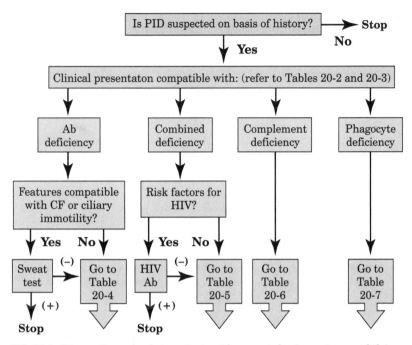

FIG. 20-1. Diagnostic approach to patients with suspected primary immunodeficiency disease.

defined by immunoglobulin levels two standard deviations below the mean for age. Some investigators recommend measuring IgG subclasses.

Saline isohemagglutinins (anti-A, anti-B) are used to assess IgM function. Isohemagglutinins are normally lacking in persons with blood type AB and are unreliable in infants <6 mos of age or in individuals who have received IV gammaglobulin (IVIG) within 30 days.

Antibody response to immunization is an example of a functional test of the immune system. Pre- and post-immunization antibody titers should be measured 3–4 wks apart. Pneumococcal polysaccharide vaccination (e.g., Pneumovax 23) is more useful for detection of impaired antibody production than protein-conjugated polysaccharide vaccines (e.g., Hib-Tetanus or Hib-Diphtheria conjugates), though it is advisable to measure responses to both polysaccharide and protein-conjugated vaccines (refer to Appendix B for reference lab values). Antibody responses to carbohydrate antigens are typically poor in children <2 yrs old.

TABLE 20-4. LAB EVALUATION FOR SUSPECTED ANTIBODY DEFICIENCY

Quantitative immunoglobulins

Pre- and post-immunization antibody titers for pneumococcal polysaccharide vaccine, *Hemophilus influenzae* type b, diptheria, and tetanus toxoid

Isohemagglutinins (anti-A, anti-B)

TABLE 20-5. LAB EVALUATION SCHEME FOR SUSPECTED COMBINED IMMUNODEFICIENCY

CBC with differential

T and B lymphocyte subsets (Immune competence panel)[a]

Delayed type hypersensitivity skin tests

Lymphocyte transformation to mitogen and antigen stimulation[a]

[a]Refer to Appendix B for reference lab values.

Lab Evaluation for Suspected Combined Immunodeficiency

See Table 20-5 for a complete list.

Rule out HIV infection before proceeding with other lab testing (see Fig. 20-1).

CBC may indicate lymphopenia. Total lymphocyte count should be >1,200 cells/mm^3. Because T cells make up approximately 75% of the total lymphocyte count, lymphopenia typically implies a decreased number of T cells.

Delayed type hypersensitivity (DTH) skin tests are functional tests of cell-mediated immunity. Only four antigens intended for assessing a person's ability to elicit a DTH response have been standardized for this use by the Mantoux procedure: tuberculin, coccidioidin, histoplasmin, and mumps. However, only a very small proportion of the population will react to tuberculin, and sensitivity to coccidioidin and histoplasmin is restricted to endemic regions. In large trials conducted at Army medical centers, mumps, *Candida*, and tetanus toxoid produced the highest proportion of positive skin tests, although only mumps is standardized for anergy testing [4].

T and B lymphocyte subsets (CD3, CD4, CD8) and *in vitro* **responses to mitogens** should be measured by a lab that provides age-matched normal control values (see Appendix B).

Lab Evaluation for Suspected Complement Deficiency

See Table 20-6 for a complete list.

Total hemolytic complement (CH50) (refer to Appendix B for reference lab values) approaches zero in individuals with deficiency of any of the classic complement pathway components (except for C9).

C3-deficient individuals exhibit the most severe form of complement deficiency due to the pivotal role of C3 in both the classic and alternative complement pathways.

Lab Evaluation for Suspected Phagocyte Deficiency

See Table 20-7 for a complete list.

CBC (refer to Appendix B for reference lab values) may reveal leukocytosis, a sign of leukocyte adhesion defect. Serial CBCs are necessary to establish a diagnosis of cyclic neutropenia.

The **quantitative flow cytometry respiratory burst assay** or the nitroblue tetrazolium test to demonstrate failure of the normal respiratory burst in chronic granulatomous disease.

TABLE 20-6. LAB EVALUATION FOR SUSPECTED COMPLEMENT DEFICIENCY

Serum total hemolytic complement (CH50)

Serum C3

Serum C4

TABLE 20-7. LAB EVALUATION FOR SUSPECTED PHAGOCYTE DEFICIENCY

(Serial) CBC with differential

Nitroblue tetrazolium test or quantitative flow cytometry respiratory burst assay

Selected Primary Immunodeficiency Diseases

It is beyond the scope of this book to provide an exhaustive review of the clinical and lab features of PID. Table 20-8 summarizes the immunologic profile and genetic defects associated with various PIDs.

IgA Deficiency

IgA deficiency is the **most common PID**, affecting 1:500–1:700 otherwise healthy individuals. Diagnostic criteria for selective IgA deficiency are outlined in Table 20-9.

Levels of other immunoglobulin classes may be elevated. IgG subclasses may be abnormally low (refer to Appendix B). Antibody function, measured by response to vaccines, is typically normal, as is cell-mediated immunity. The disease is more prevalent among persons with recurrent infections, allergy, autoimmune disorders, and certain GI disorders, such as celiac disease. IgA deficiency may be inherited in either an autosomal dominant or autosomal recessive fashion.

The clinical expression of IgA deficiency ranges from recurrent sinopulmonary or GI infections to no symptoms. *An estimated one-third of patients with IgA deficiency have serum IgE antibodies to IgA that can cause anaphylaxis during transfusion of blood products or IVIG.* **Treatment** of IgA deficiency is supportive, with antimicrobial therapy as needed and treatment of autoimmune disorders. IVIG may be considered for patients with combined IgA and IgG subclass deficiency, with the understanding that there is a risk of anaphylaxis due to trace amounts of IgA contained in IVIG.

Common Variable Immunodeficiency

Common variable immunodeficiency is **a heterogeneous disorder** characterized by recurrent bacterial infections, severe hypogammaglobulinemia, and diminished antibody responses. It typically affects older children or adults and is classically diagnosed in the second and third decades of life. Clinical manifestations include recurrent sinopulmonary infections, bronchiectasis, malabsorption, and diarrhea (usually associated with *Giardia lamblia* infection). Some patients have a respiratory tract colonization with *Mycoplasma* or *Ureaplasma* organisms. Patients also have a *higher-than-normal frequency of autoimmune disease* (e.g., pernicious anemia, hemolytic anemia, polyarticular arthritis, SLE-like syndromes), and lymphoreticular malignancy. Physical exam may reveal diminished lymphoid and tonsillar tissue, though there may be signs of lymphoid hypertrophy in the form of lymphadenopathy, splenomegaly, and intestinal nodular lymphoid hyperplasia. Serum IgG and IgA levels are usually low, and most antibody responses are poor or absent. T cell function is also impaired in some patients. Treatment is supportive, including IVIG.

Treatment

General guidelines for treatment of PID are

- Pathogen **avoidance**.
- Early and judicious use of **antibiotics**. Consider fungal, mycobacterial, viral, or protozoan pathogens early in management if infection is refractory to antibiotics.
- **IVIG** is the cornerstone of management of PID due to antibody deficiency.

  1. **Mechanism of action**. Commercially available preparations contain IgG antibodies in concentrations sufficient to serve as replacement therapy for IgG as well as trace amounts of IgA and IgM.

TABLE 20-8. IMMUNOLOGIC PROFILES AND GENETIC DEFECTS OF SELECTED PRIMARY IMMUNODEFICIENCY DISEASES

General category	Disorder	T cell levels	B cell levels	Ig levels	Defect
Combined T and B cell deficiencies	gamma chain deficiency	Low	Normal to high	Low	Defect of gamma chain of receptors for IL-2, IL-4, IL-7, IL-9, IL-15
	Jak 3 kinase deficiency	Low	Normal to high	Low	Jak 3 intracellular signaling kinase defect
	Adenosine deaminase deficiency	Progressive decrease	Progressive decrease	Low	Build-up of toxic purine pathway intermediates in lymphocytes
	Purine nucleoside phosphorylase deficiency	Progressive decrease	Normal	Normal or low	Build-up of toxic purine pathway intermediates in T lymphocytes
	MHC II deficiency (Bare Lymphocyte syndrome)	Low CD4	Normal	Normal or low	Mutation in factors controlling MHC II gene expression
	ZAP-70 kinase deficiency	Low CD8	Normal	Normal	Thymocyte intracellular kinase defect, blocked maturation of T cells
	Recombinase activating gene (RAG-1, RAG-2) deficiency	Low	Absent	Absent	Failure of T cell or B cell receptor rearrangement, blocked lymphocyte development
	Reticular dysgenesis	Low	Low	Low	Unknown bone marrow stem cell defect
	Omenn syndrome	Low	Low	Low	Missense mutation in RAG-1 or RAG-2 resulting in partial V-D-J recombination activity [5]
	DiGeorge syndrome	Normal to low	Normal	Normal to low	Embryologic defect of thymic development; variably associated defects of heart, parathyroid, facial development

continued

TABLE 20-8. CONTINUED

General category	Disorder	T cell levels	B cell levels	Ig levels	Defect
Antibody deficiencies	X-linked agammaglobulinemia	Normal	Very low to absent	Low to absent	Defect of B cell–specific Bruton tyrosine kinase
	X-linked hyper-IgM syndrome	Normal	Normal	Normal to high IgM, low IgA and IgG	Defect of CD40 ligand causing failure of B cell isotype switch
	Mu heavy chain deficiency	Normal	Absent	Absent	Defect of cell surface mu chain expression
	IgA deficiency and IgG subclass deficiency	Normal	Normal	One or more immunoglobulin types low	Unknown defects in B cell isotype expression, IgG subclass deficiencies associated with immunoglobulin heavy or light chain gene deletions
	Common variable immunodeficiency	Normal	Normal or low	Low (variable)	Unkown late-onset variable defects in B and T cell function and regulation
	Transient hypogammaglobulinemia of infancy	Normal	Normal	IgG low, IgA low or normal, IgM normal	Delayed onset of IgG synthesis; cause unknown
Other distinctive syndromes	Wiskott-Aldrich syndrome	Normal to low	Normal	Normal (some low IgM)	Defect of WASP gene involved in cytoskeleton, sparse small platelets, eczema
	Ataxia telangiectasia	Normal	Normal	Low	DNA repair defect in ATM gene; ataxia, progressive neurodegeneration; cancer; radiation sensitivity
	Bloom syndrome	Normal	Normal	Selective IgM deficiency (commonly)	DNA repair defect in BLM gene, progressive neurodegeneration, cancer, radiation sensitivity

Disorder				Description
Hyper-IgE syndrome (Job syndrome)	Normal	Normal	High IgE	Unknown, susceptibility to cutaneous boils and lung abscesses
X-linked lymphoproliferative syndrome (Duncan's syndrome)	Normal	Normal	Normal initially with progressive loss over time	Failure to resolve Epstein-Barr virus infections associated with lymphoproliferation and, ultimately, hypogammaglobulinemia
Cartilage-hair hypoplasia	Low	Normal	Normal	Short-limbed dwarfism associated with cellular immunodeficiency
Phagocyte disorders				
Chronic granulomatous disease	Normal	Normal	Normal	Impaired killing of ingested organisms due to defects of neutrophil cytochrome oxidase system
Leukocyte adhesion deficiency	Normal	Normal	Normal	Defects of leukocyte surface proteins required for adherence, migration, and phagocytosis (CD18, LAD type I)
Chediak-Higashi syndrome	Normal	Normal	Normal	Defect of *CHM* gene causing faulty lysosomal assembly, giant cytoplasmic granules, impaired neutrophil function
Complement disorders				
Individual component deficiencies	Normal	Normal	Normal	C1, C2, C4, and C3 deficiencies associated with autoimmunity and pyogenic infections; C5-9 and properdin deficiencies associated with recurrent neisserial infections

IL, interleukin.
Table adapted from Puck JM. Primary immunodeficiency diseases. *JAMA* 1997;278(22):1838–1839.

TABLE 20-9. DIAGNOSIS OF IgA DEFICIENCY

Serum IgA level less than 5 mg/dL

Normal levels of other Ig classes (IgG, IgM, IgD, IgE)

Normal or nearly normal cellular immunity

2. **Dosage.** Usual starting dose is 300–400 mg/kg/mo. Trough serum IgG levels (target >500 mg/dL or low normal) measured 4 wks after IVIG infusion are used to guide dosage and frequency.
3. **Adverse effects** include fever, chills, nausea, vomiting, and back pain. Severe anaphylactoid reactions may occur (possibly due to trace amounts of IgA in the IVIG). Aseptic meningitis is a rare adverse effect.

- **Stem cell transplantation** has been used to correct the underlying immune defects in severe combined immunodeficiency (SCID) and Wiskott-Aldrich syndrome. Research is underway in other PIDs.
- **Gene therapy** and replacement enzyme therapy are investigational.
- **Precautions**

1. **Blood products** may elicit life-threatening graft-versus-host disease in patients with cellular immunodeficiency.
2. **Live virus vaccines** should not be given to patients with PID or their family members.

KEY POINTS

- IgA deficiency is the most common PID.
- Most PIDs are due to antibody deficiencies.
- Types of infections and etiologic agents are powerful clues to the subtype of PID.

SUGGESTED READING AND WEB SITES

National Institute of Allergy and Infectious Diseases website: http://www.niaid.nih.gov/publications/pid.htm.

Paul ME, Shearer WT. The patient with 'too many infections': diagnostic approach. In: *Current clinical practice: allergic diseases: diagnosis and treatment*, 2nd ed. Totowa, NJ: Humana Press, 2000:445–459.

Polmar SH, Kemp ME. Immunodeficiency diseases. In: *Allergy: theory and practice*, 2nd ed. Philadelphia: WB Saunders, 1992:103–128.

Puck JM. Primary immunodeficiency diseases. *JAMA* 1997;278(22):1838–1839.

REFERENCES

1. Genes and mechanisms underlying primary immunodeficiency. NIH Guide, Volume 26, Number 29, August 29, 1997.
2. Workshop on registries for primary immunodeficiency diseases. NIAID and the Office of Rare Diseases, NIH, November 19, 1996.
3. Stiehm ER, Chin TW, Haas A, et al. Infectious complications of the primary immunodeficiencies. *Clin Immunol Immunopathol* 1986;40(1):69–86.
4. CDC. Purified protein derivative (PPD)-tuberculin anergy and HIV infection: guidelines for anergy testing and management of anergic persons at risk of tuberculosis. *MMWR Morb Mortal Wkly Rep* 1991;40:27–33.
5. Wada T, Takei K, Kudo M, et al. Characterization of immune function and analysis of RAG gene mutations in Omenn syndrome and related disorders. *Clin Exp Immunol* 2000;119(1):148–155.

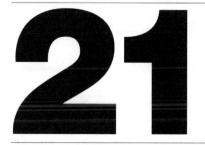

Allergen Immunotherapy

Jill A. Poole

INTRODUCTION

Allergen immunotherapy (IT) is the administration of increasing doses of allergen extract to alleviate symptoms associated with the causative allergen. It was first used by Noon and Freeman to treat hay fever (allergic rhinitis) in 1911 [1,2]. Today it is used in allergic rhinitis, allergic asthma, and stinging-insect hypersensitivity. Standardized extracts should be used when available. IT should only be performed by a specialist trained in allergy.

MECHANISM

The mechanism [3,4] of action of IT is unknown. One current theory is that immune modulation of the immune system shifts the T cell phenotype from a Th2 towards a Th1 predominance. A complex cytokine cascade is thought to govern inflammatory cell recruitment involved in immediate and late-phase inflammatory reactions (Fig. 21-1).

Studies have shown that IT leads to

- Blunting of the usual seasonal rise in IgE antibodies.
- Increase in serum IgG antibodies with change in subclasses (increased IgG1 and IgG4).
- Down-regulation of the cellular and inflammatory mediators of allergic response.

  - Decrease in platelet activating factor and histamine-releasing factor levels.
  - Down-regulation of the low-affinity IgE receptor (FCeRIIB).
  - Decrease in mast cell and eosinophil numbers in secretions.

- Up-regulation of the counter-regulatory cytokines expressed by Th1 phenotype.

CLINICAL EFFICACY [3,8]

The clinical efficacy of IT in allergic rhinitis has been well documented, and IT has been shown to improve symptoms, reduce medications, and provide long-term benefits even after cessation of therapy [6,11,12]. Allergen-specific IT has the potential to alter the natural course of allergic disease [5]. Long-term benefits of >3 yrs after discontinuation of therapy in patients with allergic rhinitis have been documented [6]. Preliminary results from a preventive allergy treatment study suggest that treating children with allergic rhinitis with IT protects them from developing asthma [7].

The quality of the extract used for successful IT is critical. The World Health Organization (WHO) has endorsed the use of standardized extracts in IT [10]. Techniques for immunologic standardization have allowed the preparation of standard extracts for a number of important aeroallergens. On the other hand, the FDA has standardized allergen extracts based on their total biologic activity. Using either method, allergen extracts are commercially available for many allergens [3].

Achieving optimal target doses of the causative allergen is also critical for IT to be successful. Table 21-1 provides recommended maintenance doses set forth by the joint task force for allergen immunotherapy practice parameters [25]. However,

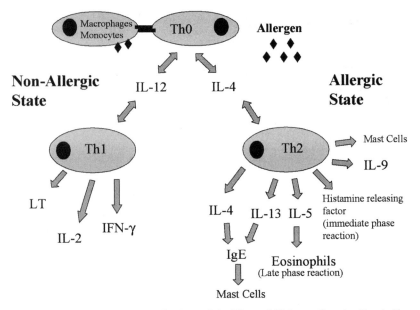

FIG. 21-1. Simplified schematic diagram of the Th1 and Th2 paradigm in allergic diseases. The Th2 profile is associated with the allergic state and humoral immune responses, whereas the Th1 profile is associated with cellular responses and a downregulation in allergic responses. Immunotherapy is thought to shift the T cell phenotype from Th2 toward Th1. A representation of cytokines involved in this is shown. LT, lymphotoxin; Th0, undifferentiated T-helper cell.

TABLE 21-1 ALLERGEN IMMUNOTHERAPY RECOMMENDED MAINTENANCE DOSES

Allergen	Dose, standardized units	Dose, major allergen	Maintenance concentrate, wt/vol[a]
Dermatophagoides pteronyssinus	600 AU	7–12 μg, Der p1	NA
Dermatophagoides farinae	2,000 AU	10 μg, Der f1	NA
Cat	2,000–3,000 BAU	11–17 μg, Fel d1	NA
Grass (e.g., timothy)	4,000 BAU	7 μg, Phl p5	NA
Short ragweed (standardized)	NA	6–24 μg, Amb a1	1:100–1:30
Other pollen (nonstandardized)	NA	ND	1:100–1:30
Fungi/mold (nonstandardized)	NA	ND	1:100–1:50

AU, allergy unit; BAU, bioequivalent allergy unit; NA, not applicable; ND, not determined.
[a]Based on a maintenance injection of 0.5 ml.
Reprinted from reference 25, with permission.

the most efficacious dose of allergen is not well characterized for most allergens, and, therefore, the recommended doses are not solidly supported by data. Clearly, more studies are needed to define what constitutes an effective allergen extract dose [9]. An excellent review of dosing considerations in allergen IT can be found in reference 3.

CLINICAL INDICATIONS FOR IMMUNOTHERAPY

IT is indicated for allergic rhinitis/conjunctivitis, allergic reactions to stinging insects, and allergic asthma. It is not indicated for food or drug allergy, urticaria, angioedema, or atopic dermatitis [10].

Before starting IT the following criteria should be met:

- Demonstration that the disease is IgE-mediated, which is most reliably done by skin prick testing.
- Attempts to avoid allergen have either been less than successful or impossible.
- Pharmacotherapy (antihistamines, decongestants, antileukotrienes, topical corticosteroids) has not successfully controlled symptoms.

Indications for IT (any one of the following):

- Insufficient symptom control with antihistamines, decongestants, topical corticosteroids, and/or antileukotrienes.
- Undesirable side effects of pharmacotherapy.
- Desire to reduce long-term pharmacologic treatment.
- Patients with allergic asthma with mild-moderate disease: $FEV_1 > 70\%$ of predicted value on adequate pharmacologic treatment. [IT is contraindicated if peak expiratory flow rate (PEFR) $<70\%$ due to an increased risk of death from anaphylaxis or bronchospasm.]

Specific Clinical Indications for Immunotherapy in Allergic Rhinitis

Commonly cited reasons for using IT in allergic rhinitis [10,25]:

- To prevent symptoms and improve quality of life.
- To reduce ongoing expenses for noncurative medication.
- To reduce side effects of antihistamines and decongestants.
- To reduce development/aggravation of allergic asthma.
- To reduce comorbidity due to recurrent sinusitis/otitis.
- To improve on the limited efficacy of allergen avoidance.

Specific Clinical Indications for Immunotherapy in Allergic Asthma

In the past, the role of IT in allergic asthma had been controversial, but two large meta-analyses confirmed effectiveness of IT in treating mild to moderate allergic asthma compared to placebo [13,14]. These studies demonstrated that patients treated with IT had reductions in allergen-specific bronchial hyperresponsiveness, medication requirements, and overall symptoms. Therefore, IT has been endorsed by the WHO for the treatment of mild to moderate allergic asthma [10].

Fig. 21-2 provides an algorithm of when IT may be initiated in the treatment of mild to moderate allergic asthma. As shown, there are two basic strategies. Starting IT early in the course of allergic asthma may lead to decreased use of medications and, perhaps, even an alteration in the natural course of the disease, as discussed in the section Clinical Efficacy.

Specific Clinical Indications for Immunotherapy in Insect-Sting Hypersensitivity

The efficacy of IT is clearly efficacious in venom hypersensitivity. IT is indicated for patients with a history of anaphylaxis from venom [15] (see Chap. 13, Anaphylaxis).

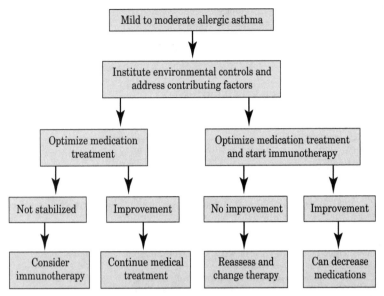

FIG. 21-2. When to initiate immunotherapy in mild to moderate allergic asthma. There are two basic strategies. The first involves reserving immunotherapy for only those patients who do not stabilize despite institution of environmental controls and medications. The second involves early institution of immunotherapy. The advantage of the latter is reducing medication requirements and perhaps altering the natural course of the disease.

TREATMENT

- Allergen IT needs to be individualized to the patient.
- IT is traditionally given at weekly intervals while increasing the dose to maintenance therapy.
- Rush protocols (injections given daily) and cluster protocols (multiple injections/day) are used more commonly in Europe. The exception is for insect-sting hypersensitivity, in which rush protocols are used more commonly.
- A sample schedule for perennial aqueous IT is given in Appendix C.
- Allergen extract concentrations can be expressed as a weight per volume ratio, protein nitrogen unit, or, the biologically active measure, in allergen units.
- IT should be prepared and administered under the supervision of a trained allergy specialist.
- The goal is to attain the highest tolerated dose; normally 6–12 μg per injection of the major allergen is required.
- A physician needs to be immediately available with proper equipment on hand to treat anaphylaxis.
- The favored injection site is the outer aspect of the upper arm between the deltoid and triceps muscles.
- Extracts are administered SC.
- The patient should be observed for at least 20 mins after the injection, per the WHO and American Academy of Allergy, Asthma, and Immunology guidelines. However, a 30-min observation period is used by many allergists.

Duration of Treatment

Three to 5 yrs of therapy is generally given; however, the actual length of time for treatment is unclear. The recommendation of 3–5 yrs is based on data from venom hypersensitivity and only one study of a single seasonal allergen (grass); clearly, further studies need to be performed [6]. If symptoms are well controlled after this time, IT may be stopped. Symptoms will recur within 1–2 years after cessation of IT in some patients, and in these patients, IT is often restarted. In any patient, if there is no apparent clinical benefit from IT after 1–2 yrs, IT should be discontinued.

Side Effects and Risks [10,16]

Local reactions are common. Significant local reactions are identified as an immediate redness and swelling with wheal >2 cm in diameter, or wheal lasting >24 hrs. Local reactions should be treated with oral antihistamine and local application of cold packs. After the occurrence of a local reaction, the current practice is to continue IT but to reduce the amount of allergenic extract to the previously tolerated dose. Reviewing the technique of administration may also be beneficial. For allergic rhinitis and asthma, premedication is not routinely used. However, in venom IT, studies suggest that initial antihistamine premedication might actually increase the efficacy of venom IT [17].

Systemic reaction/anaphylaxis is rare. Generalized erythema, urticaria, pruritus, angioedema, bronchospasm, laryngeal edema, shock, and cardiac arrest have all been reported. These reactions should be treated with IM aqueous epinephrine (0.3–0.5 cc of 1:1,000). To limit systemic absorption of the antigen, a tourniquet should be placed above the injection site and released every 15 mins. Optionally, epinephrine, 0.1–0.3 cc, may also be given at the injection site to further delay absorption of the antigen. Because of its more rapid onset, the preferred antihistamine is diphenhydramine (Benadryl), and it is given IV or IM. Replacement of intravascular volume may be required as well. IV hydrocortisone (5 mg/kg) may be used for severe systemic reactions; however, corticosteroids have limited effect in the immediate response. In general, they are used to prevent a late-phase response, which may occur 4–12 hrs after the initial response and can be as severe. A trained physician with proper emergency resuscitation equipment needs to be immediately available to administer life-saving treatment.

A fatal systemic reaction occurs in approximately one out of every 2 million doses of IT administered annually [16,18]. Each patient should know that there are risks involved in receiving IT. The WHO recommends that patients wait in the office at least 20 mins after receiving an injection. A longer waiting period is necessary if using rush IT or if the patient has unstable asthma, a high degree of sensitivity, or seasonal exacerbation of symptoms or if the patient is on a beta-blocker [10]. A physician needs to be immediately available at all times to perform emergency treatment if necessary.

Special Considerations and Relative Contraindications [10]

- Ongoing treatment with a beta-adrenergic blocker is a relative contraindication. Patients receiving beta-blockers (typically patients with cardiovascular disease, hypertension, or migraine headaches) are at increased risk for a severe anaphylactic reaction that may be resistant to epinephrine administration. Decisions to initiate IT in such patients must be carefully evaluated.
- IT is contraindicated in patients with epinephrine sensitivity, because these patients cannot tolerate life-saving treatment.
- IT is contraindicated in allergic asthma patients with PEFR <70% as risk of severe bronchospasm is increased.
- IT is relatively contraindicated in the very young and old.
- It may be necessary to hold or reduce dosage during a particularly bad pollen season.
- Do not generally give injections to a patient with a fever, an asthmatic with upper respiratory infection, a wheezing patient, or a patient with significantly reduced pulmonary function tests (PEFR <70%).
- Strenuous exercise should be avoided after an injection.
- Pregnant women can continue IT at lower doses than normal. Do not initiate IT in a pregnant woman, because the potential risk to the fetus of using epinephrine for anaphylaxis treatment is too high.

POTENTIAL REASONS FOR FAILURE OF IMMUNOTHERAPY

- Environmental controls are inadequate or insufficient.
- Significant or contributing allergen not recognized and included in IT regimen.
- Inadequate doses of major allergen in preparation (normally need 6–12 μg of the major allergen to be successful).
- New allergies develop during treatment course.
- Original causative allergen is misdiagnosed.
- Patient has unrealistic expectations.

FUTURE DIRECTIONS

Future research in allergy IT is continuing to grow rapidly. One goal is to modify current IT to reduce side effects while enhancing immunogenicity. DNA vaccines using DNA immunostimulatory sequences (the so-called CpG motif) combined with purified allergen have reduced anaphylactic reactions while increasing the immune response in experimental animal studies [19,20]. In addition, peptide IT (isolated peptide fragments, epitopes), which works by maintaining T-cell reactivity without cross-linking cell-bound IgE, is being studied and has the possibility of reducing the chances of triggering an allergic response while still providing the benefits of traditional IT [21].

Another direction of research is into novel immune modulation therapies that act by promoting a shift of the immune response from a Th2 toward a Th1 predominance. Investigational research strategies can be found in a review article [22]. Therapies that may reach FDA approval soon include monoclonal anti-IgE[23] and a soluble IL-4 receptor protein that antagonizes IL-4 activity [24].

KEY POINTS

- Mechanism is unknown, but may involve immune modulation by shifting Th2 to Th1 phenotype.
- Allergy IT should be used when pharmacotherapy and allergen avoidance fail to control symptoms.
- Contraindications to IT are in allergic asthma patients with PEFR <70%. Special considerations are needed for pregnant women, patients on beta-blockers, and patients with concurrent illness.
- Treatment needs to be tailored for the individual, with appropriate concentrations of allergens for approximately a 3–5 yr duration.

REFERENCES

1. Noon L. Prophylactic inoculation against hay fever. *Lancet* 1911;1:1572–1573.
2. Freeman J. Further observations of the treatment of hay fever by hypodermic inoculations of pollen vaccine. *Lancet* 1911;2:814–817.
3. Creticos PS. Immunotherapy of allergic diseases. In: Rich RR, ed. *Clinical immunology principles and practice*. St. Louis: Mosby, 1996:2002–2018.
4. Creticos PS. The consideration of immunotherapy in the treatment of allergic asthma. *Ann Allergy Asthma Immunol* 2001;87(Suppl):13–27.
5. Bousquet J, Demoly P, Michel FB. Specific immunotherapy in rhinitis and asthma. *Ann Allergy Asthma Immunol* 2001;87(Suppl):38–42.
6. Durham SR, Walker SM, Varga EM, et al. Long-term clinical efficacy of grass-pollen immunotherapy. *N Engl J Med* 1999;342:468–475.
7. Jacobsen L. Preventive aspects of immunotherapy: prevention for children at risk of developing asthma. *Ann Allergy Asthma Immunol* 2001;87(Suppl):43–46.
8. Weber RW. Immunotherapy with allergens. *JAMA* 1997;278:1881–1887.
9. Nelson HS. The use of standardized extracts in allergen immunotherapy. *J Allergy Clin Immunol* 2000;106:41–45.

10. Theodoropoulos DS, Lockey RF. Allergen immunotherapy: guidelines, update, and recommendations of the World Health Organization. *Allergy Asthma Proc* 2000;21:159–168.
11. Lowell FC, Franklin W. A double-blind study of the effectiveness and specificity of injection therapy in ragweed hay fever. *N Engl J Med* 1965;273:675–679.
12. Varney VA, Gaga M, Frew AJ, et al. Usefulness of immunotherapy in ragweed hay fever. *N Engl J Med* 1965;273:265–269.
13. Abramson MJ, Puy RM, Weiner JM. Immunotherapy in asthma: an updated systematic review. *Allergy* 1999;54:1022–1041.
14. Abramson MJ, Puy RM, Weiner JM. Is allergen immunotherapy effective in asthma? *Am J Respir Crit Care Med* 1995;151:969–974.
15. Hunt KJ, Valentine MD, Sobotka AK, et al. A controlled trial of immunotherapy in insect hypersensitivity. *N Engl J Med* 1978;299:157–161.
16. Lockey RF, Nicoara-Kasti GL, Theodoropoulos DS, Bukantz SC. Systemic reactions and fatalities associated with allergen immunotherapy. *Ann Allergy Asthma Immunol* 2001;87(Suppl):47–55.
17. Muller UR. New developments in the diagnosis and treatment of hymenoptera venom. *Int Arch Allergy Immunol* 2001;124:447–553.
18. Steward GE, Lockey RF. Systemic reactions from allergen immunotherapy. *J Allergy Clinical Immunol* 1992;90:567–579.
19. Tighe H, Takabayashi K, Schwartz D, et al. Conjugation of immunostimulatory DNA to the short ragweed allergen AMB al enhances its immunogenicity and reduces its allergenicity. *J Allergy Clin Immunol* 2000;106:124–134.
20. Horner A, Nguyen MD, Ronaghy A, et al. DNA-based vaccination reduces the risk of lethal anaphylactic hypersensitivity in mice. *J Allergy Clin Immunol* 2000;106:349–356.
21. Haselden BM, Kay AB, Larche M. Peptide-mediated immune responses in specific immunotherapy. *Int Arch Allergy Immunol* 2000;122:229–237.
22. Woodruff PG, Fahy JV. Asthma: prevalence, pathogenesis, and prospects for novel therapies. *JAMA* 2001;286:395–398.
23. Milgrom H, Fick RB, Su JQ, et al. Treatment of allergic asthma with monoclonal anti-IgE antibody. *N Engl J Med* 1999;341:1966–1973.
24. Borish LC, Nelson HS, Corren J, et al. Efficacy of soluble IL-4 receptor for the treatment of adults with asthma. *J Allergy Clin Immunol* 2001;107:963–970.
25. Li JT, Lockey RF, Bernstein IL, et al., for the Joint Task Force on Practice Parameters. Allergen immunotherapy: a practice parameter. *Ann Allergy, Asthma, Immunol* 2003;90:S1–S140.

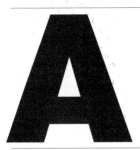

Drugs Commonly Used in Allergy and Asthma

Anne C. Graff and
Diane R. Klueppel

TABLE A-1. ANTIHISTAMINES

Generic name	Brand name(s)	Adult dosage
First generation		
Diphenhydramine	Benadryl	25–50 q4–6h prn
Chlorpheniramine	Chlor-Trimeton, others	4 mg q4–6h prn
Brompheniramine	Dimetapp, others	4 mg q4–6h prn
Hydroxyzine	Atarax, Vistaril	25–100 mg qd–qid prn
Second generation		
Cetirizine	Zyrtec	5 or 10 mg qd
Fexofenadine	Allegra	60 mg bid or 180 mg qd
Loratadine	Claritin	10 mg qd
Desloratadine	Clarinex	5 mg qd

TABLE A-2. INTRANASAL CORTICOSTEROIDS

Generic name	Brand name(s)	Adult dosage
Beclomethasone dipropionate	Beconase AQ	42 μg/spray: 1–2 sprays each nostril bid
	Vancenase AQ	84 μg/spray: 1–2 sprays each nostril qd
Budesonide	Rhinocort Aqua	32 μg/spray: 1–4 sprays each nostril qd
Flunisolide	Nasalide, Nasarel	25 μg/spray: 2 sprays each nostril bid
Fluticasone propionate	Flonase	50 μg/spray: 2 sprays each nostril qd or 1 spray each nostril bid
Mometasone furoate	Nasonex	50 μg/spray: 2 sprays each nostril qd
Triamcinolone acetonide	Nasacort AQ	55 μg/spray: 2 sprays each nostril qd

TABLE A-3. INTRANASAL ANTIHISTAMINES

Generic name	Brand name(s)	Adult dosage
Azelastine	Astelin	137 μg/spray: 2 sprays each nostril bid

TABLE A-4. OTHER INTRANASAL PREPARATIONS

Ipratropium bromide	Atrovent	0.03% (21 μg/spray): 2 sprays each nostril bid–tid
		0.06% (42 μg/spray): 2 sprays each nostril tid–qid

TABLE A-5. OPHTHALMIC ANTIALLERGY PREPARATIONS

Generic name	Brand name(s)	Adult dosage
Antihistamines/decongestants		
Naphazoline + pheniramine	Naphcon-A	1 gtt bid–qid prn
Naphazoline + antazoline	Vasocon-A	1 gtt qid prn
Antihistamines		
Levocabastine 0.05%	Livostin	1 gtt qid prn
Emedastine 0.05%	Emadine	1 gtt qid prn
Azelastine 0.05%	Optivar	1 gtt bid
Antihistamines/mast cell stabilizer		
Olopatadine 0.1%	Patanol	1 gtt bid
Ketotifen fumarate 0.025%	Zaditor	1 gtt q8–12h
Mast cell stabilizers		
Lodoxamide tromethamine 0.1%	Alomide	1 gtt qid
Nedocromil sodium 2%	Alocril	1 gtt bid
Cromolyn sodium 4%	Crolom, Opticrom	1 gtt q4–6h
Pemirolast potassium 0.1%	Alamast	1 gtt qid
NSAIDs		
Ketorolac tromethamine 0.5%	Acular	1 gtt qid
Diclofenac sodium 0.1%	Voltaren	1 gtt qid
Steroids		
Prednisolone acetate 0.12%	Pred Mild	1 gtt bid–qid
Loteprednol etabonate 0.2%	Alrex	1 gtt qid
Loteprednol etabonate 0.5%	Lotemax	1 gtt qid

TABLE A-6. INHALED BETA$_2$-AGONISTS

Generic name	Brand name(s)	Adult dosage
Short acting		
Albuterol sulfate	Proventil, Ventolin	Nebulized (5 mg/mL): 2.5 mg q6–8h prn
		MDI (90 μg/puff): 2 puffs q4–6h prn
Levalbuterol	Xopenex	Nebulized: 0.63–1.25 mg tid prn
Pirbuterol acetate	Maxair, Maxair Autohaler	MDI or Autohaler (200 μg/puff): 2 puffs q4–6h prn
Long acting		
Salmeterol	Serevent	MDI (21 μg/puff): 2 puffs q12h
	Serevent Diskus	Dry-powder inhaler (50 μg/inhalation): 1 inhalation q12h
Formoterol fumarate	Foradil Aerolizer	Dry-powder inhaler (12 μg/inhalation): 1 inhalation q12h

TABLE A-7. INHALED CORTICOSTEROIDS

Generic name	Brand name(s)	Adult dosage
Beclomethasone dipropionate	Beclovent, Vanceril, Vanceril DS	MDI (42 μg/puff,): 2 puffs tid–qid or 4 puffs bid (84 μg/puff): 2 puffs bid
Budesonide	Pulmicort Turbu-haler	Dry-powder inhaler (200 μg/inhalation): 200–800 μg bid
Flunisolide	Aerobid, Aerobid-M	MDI (250 μg/puff): 2–4 puffs bid
Fluticasone prop-rionate	Flovent	MDI (44, 110, 220 μg/puff): 88–880 μg bid
		Dry-powder inhaler (50, 100, 250 μg/inhalation): 100–1,000 μg bid
Triamcinolone acetonide	Azmacort	MDI (100 μg/puff): 2 puffs tid–qid or 4 puffs bid

Note: Common dosages are reported and may vary with the severity of disease. Inhaled corticosteroids are expressed using low dose recommendations as reported in the 1997 NIH/NHLBI guidelines for the management of asthma.

TABLE A-7A. ESTIMATED COMPARATIVE DAILY DOSAGES FOR INHALED CORTICOSTEROIDS (ADULTS)

Drug	Low dose	Medium dose	High dose
Beclomethasone dipropionate	168–504 μg	504–840 μg	>840 μg
42 μg/puff	4–12 puffs	12–20 puffs	>20 puffs
84 μg/puff	2–6 puffs	6–10 puffs	>10 puffs
Budesonide *Turbuhaler*	200–400 μg	400–600 μg	>600 μg
200 μg/dose	1–2 inhalations	2–3 inhalations	>3 inhalations
Flunisolide	500–1,000 μg	1,000–2,000 μg	>2,000 μg
250 μg/puff	2–4 puffs	4–8 puffs	>8 puffs
Fluticasone	88–264 μg	264–660 μg	>660 μg
MDI: 44, 110, 220 μg/puff	2–6 puffs (44 μg) or 2 puffs (110 μg)	2–6 puffs (110 μg)	>6 puffs (110 μg) or >3 puffs (220 μg)
DPI: 50, 100, 250 μg/puff	2–6 inhalations (50 μg)	3–6 inhalations (100 μg)	>6 inhalations (100 μg) or >2 inhalations (250 μg)
Triamcinolone acetonide	400–1,000 μg	1,000–2,000 μg	>2,000 μg
100 μg/puff	4–10 puffs	10–20 puffs	>20 puffs

Reprinted from *Guidelines for the diagnosis and management of asthma. Expert panel report 2.* National Institutes of Health. National Heart, Lung, and Blood Institute, 1997, with permission.

TABLE A-7B. PHARMACOKINETICS OF INHALED CORTICOSTEROIDS

Parameters	Beclomethasone	Budesonide	Flunisolide	Fluticasone	Triamcinolone
Absorption					
Systemic bioavailability from lungs	~20%	25%	40%	20%	21.5%
Distribution					
Vd (L/kg)	NA	4.3	1.8	3.5	1.4
Protein binding	87%	85–90%	NA	91%	~68%
Metabolism site	Liver (CYP3A)	Liver (CYP3A)	Liver	Liver (CYP3A4)	Mostly from liver, less extensively from the kidneys
Excretion					
Site	Feces, urine (<10%)	Urine (~60%) feces	Renal (50%), feces (40%)	Feces, urine (<0.02%)	Urine (~40%), feces (~60%)
$T_{1/2}$	2.8 hrs	2.8 hrs	~1.8 hrs	3.1 hrs	1.5 hrs

Vd, volume of distribution.
Reprinted from *Drug facts and comparisons*. St. Louis: Facts and Comparisons, 2001, with permission.

TABLE A-8. LEUKOTRIENE MODIFIERS

Generic name	Brand name	Adult dosage
Montelukast	Singulair	10 mg qhs
Zafirlukast	Accolate	20 mg bid
Zileuton	Zyflo	600 mg qid

TABLE A-9. OTHER ASTHMA DRUGS

Generic name	Brand name(s)	Adult dosage
Mast cell stabilizers		
Cromolyn sodium	Intal	MDI (800 μg/puff): 2 puffs qid
		Nebulizer sln (20 mg/ampule): 1 ampule qid
Nedocromil sodium	Tilade	MDI (1.75 mg/puff): 2 puffs qid
Xanthine derivatives		
Theophylline	Slo-Bid, Theo-Dur, Uniphyl, various	300–600 mg/day
Combined inhaled corticosteroid and long-acting beta-agonist		
Fluticasone + salmeterol	Advair Diskus	Dry-inhalation powder (100/250/500 μg fluticasone + 50 μg salmeterol/inhalation): 1 inhalation bid

TABLE A-10. SELECTED TOPICAL CORTICOSTEROIDS

Generic name	Brand name(s)	Vehicle
Very high potency		
Betamethasone dipropionate, augmented 0.05%	Diprolene	Ointment
Clobetasol propionate 0.05%	Temovate, others	Cream, ointment, gel
Halobetasol propionate 0.05%	Ultravate	Cream, ointment
High potency		
Amcinonide 0.1%	Cyclocort	Cream, ointment, lotion
Betamethasone dipropionate, augmented 0.05%	Diprolene AF	Cream
Betamethasone dipropionate 0.05%	Diprosone, others	Cream, ointment
Betamethasone valerate 0.1%	Betatrex	Ointment
Desoximetasone 0.05%	Topicort	Gel
Desoximetasone 0.25%	Topicort	Cream, ointment
Fluocinonide 0.05%	Lidex, others	Cream, ointment, gel
Halcinonide 0.1%	Halog, Halog-E	Cream, ointment
Triamcinolone acetonide 0.5%	Aristocort, Kenalog, others	Cream, ointment, lotion
Intermediate potency		
Betamethasone dipropionate 0.05%	Diprosone, others	Lotion
Betamethasone valerate 0.1%	Betatrex, Valisone	Cream, lotion
Desoximetasone 0.05%, 0.25%	Topicort	Cream, ointment, gel
Fluocinolone acetonide 0.025%	Synalar	Cream, ointment
Flurandrenolide 0.025%, 0.05%	Cordran	Cream, ointment, lotion
Fluticasone propionate 0.005%	Cutivate	Ointment
Fluticasone propionate 0.05%	Cutivate	Cream
Hydrocortisone butyrate 0.1%	Locoid	Cream, ointment, solution
Hydrocortisone valerate 0.2%	Westcort	Cream, ointment
Mometasone furoate 0.1%	Elocon	Cream, ointment, lotion
Triamcinolone acetonide 0.025%, 0.1%	Aristocort, Kenalog, others	Cream, ointment, lotion
Low potency		
Alclometasone dipropionate 0.05%	Aclovate	Cream, ointment
Desonide 0.05%	DesOwen	Cream, lotion, ointment
Dexamethasone sodium phosphate 0.1%	Decadron	Cream, gel
Fluocinolone acetonide 0.01%	Synalar	Cream, ointment
Hydrocortisone acetate 0.5%, 1%	Cortaid, others	Cream, ointment
Hydrocortisone 1%, 2.5%	Hytone, others	Cream, ointment, lotion

Note: Adult dosages range from qd to qid (consult labels).

TABLE A-11. GLUCOCORTICOID EQUIVALENCIES, POTENCIES, AND HALF-LIFE

Glucocorticoid	Approximate equivalent dose (mg)	Relative antiinflammatory (glucocorticoid) potency	Relative mineralocorticoid potency	Half-life Plasma (mins)	Half-life Biologic (hrs)
Short acting					
Cortisone	25	0.8	2	30	8–12
Hydrocortisone	20	1	2	80–118	8–12
Intermediate acting					
Prednisone	5	4	1	60	18–36
Prednisolone	5	4	1	115–212	18–36
Triamcinolone	4	5	0	200+	18–36
Methylprednisolone	4	5	0	78–188	18–36
Long-acting					
Dexamethasone	0.75	20–30	0	110–210	36–54
Betamethasone	0.6–0.75	20–30	0	300+	36–54

Reprinted from *Drug facts and comparisons*. St. Louis: Facts and Comparisons, 2001, with permission.

TABLE A-12. ANAPHYLAXIS KITS

Generic name	Brand name	Adult dosage
Epinephrine (1:1,000; 1 mg/mL)	EpiPen	Auto-injector (0.30 mg): 1 injection IM (0.30-mg injector recommended for most adults)
Epinephrine (1:1,000; 1 mg/mL) + chlorpheniramine	Ana-Kit	Epinephrine auto-injector containing 2 × 0.30 mg doses: 1 injection IM, repeat if needed in 10 min + 4 × 2-mg chewable tabs of chlorpheniramine (total dose = 8 mg)

SUGGESTED READING

Hebel SK, Olin BR, eds. Antihistamines. In: *Drug facts and comparisons*. St. Louis: Facts and Comparisons, 2000:699–707.

Hebel SK, Olin BR, eds. Bronchodilators. In: *Drug facts and comparisons*. St. Louis: Facts and Comparisons, 2000:643–661.

Hebel SK, Olin BR, eds. Corticosteroids: ophthalmic agents. In: *Drug facts and comparisons*. St. Louis: Facts and Comparisons, 2000:1748–1750.

Hebel SK, Olin BR, eds. Corticosteroids: respiratory inhalant products. In: *Drug facts and comparisons*. St. Louis: Facts and Comparisons, 2000:1751–1761.

Hebel SK, Olin BR, eds. Emergency kits. In: *Drug facts and comparisons*. St. Louis: Facts and Comparisons, 2000.

Hebel SK, Olin BR, eds. Intranasal steroids. In: *Drug facts and comparisons* (loose-leaf edition). St. Louis: Facts and Comparisons, 2000:673–676.

Hebel SK, Olin BR, eds. Leukotriene receptor antagonists. In: *Drug facts and comparisons*. St. Louis: Facts and Comparisons, 2000.

Hebel SK, Olin BR, eds. Leukotriene receptor inhibitors. In: *Drug facts and comparisons*. St. Louis: Facts and Comparisons, 2000.

Hebel SK, Olin BR, eds. NSAIDS: ophthalmic agents. In: *Drug facts and comparisons*. St. Louis: Facts and Comparisons, 2000:1746–1747.

Hebel SK, Olin BR, eds. Ophthalmic decongestant agents. In: *Drug facts and comparisons*. St. Louis: Facts and Comparisons, 2000:1751–1761.

Hebel SK, Olin BR, eds. Topical corticosteroids. In: *Drug facts and comparisons*. St. Louis: Facts and Comparisons, 2000:1633–1643.

Hebel SK, Olin BR, eds. Xanthine derivatives. In: *Drug facts and comparisons*. St. Louis: Facts and Comparisons, 2000.

Lacy CF, Armstrong LL, Goldman MP, Lance LL, eds. Topical corticosteroids. In: *Drug information handbook*, 8th ed. Hudson, OH: Lexi-Comp, 2000:1344–1345.

Micromedex healthcare series. Englewood, CO: Micromedex (edition expires 12/01).

NHLBI, National Asthma Education and Prevention Program, Expert Panel Report 2. *Guidelines for the diagnosis and management of asthma*. NIH Publication No. 97-4051. Bethesda, MD: U.S. Department of Health and Human Services, 1997.

USP DI, United States pharmacopeia drug information, 21st ed. Englewood, CO: Micromedex, 2001.

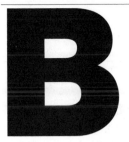

Lab Values for Selected Tests in Immunology

Robin G. Lorenz

TABLE B-1. COMPLETE BLOOD COUNT

Normal range	Adult male	Adult female
WBC	3.8–9.8 k/m^3	3.8–9.8
RBC	4.5–5.7 m/m^3	3.9–5
Hemoglobin	13.8–17.2 g/dL	12.1–15.1
Hemocrit	40.7–50.3%	36.1–44.3
Platelet	140–440 k/m^3	140–440

TABLE B-2. QUANTITATIVE IMMUNOGLOBULINS BY AGE OF PATIENT

Reference ranges	IgG (mg/dL)	IgA (mg/dL)	IgM (mg/dL)
Cord blood	636–1,660	1.4–3.8	6.3–25
1–12 mos	251–1,069	215–1,069	20–149
1–4 yrs	345–1,213	14–159	43–200
5–8 yrs	463–1,280	25–202	48–207
9 yrs–adult	608–1,572	45–312	52–352
Adult	700–1,450	70–370	30–210

TABLE B-3. QUANTITATIVE IgG SUBCLASSES BY AGE OF PATIENT

Reference ranges	IgG1	IgG2	IgG3	IgG4
0–2 yrs	170–950	21.5–440	13.4–69.4	0.4–120
2–4 yrs	290–1,065	28–315	3.5–75	0.8–90
4–6 yrs	330–1,065	56.5–345	7.5–125.6	1.8–115.5
6–8 yrs	225–1,100	42–375	9.1–106.3	0.3–138
Adult male	239.6–1083.5	123.5–548.7	27.6–134.4	8.4–888.8
Adult female	342.2–1117.8	147.6–524.6	21.1–114.2	6.9–88.8

TABLE B-4. TOTAL HEMOLYTIC COMPLEMENT

63–145 CAE units

Note: This test is now called *total complement activation.*

TABLE B-5. *HAEMOPHILUS INFLUENZAE* TYPE B ANTIBODY

>1.0 μg/mL

Note: Used to test for polysaccharide antigen-specific responses in immunized individuals. Pre-immunization levels would be <1.0 μg/mL, down to the lower limits of detection.

TABLE B-6. ANTITETANUS ANTIBODIES

>0.1 units/mL

Note: Used to test for protein antigen-specific responses in immunized individuals.

TABLE B-7. LYMPHOCYTE TRANSFORMATION TO:

Phytohemagglutinin	47,318–229,629 cpm (to measure T cell function)
Pokeweed mitogen	14,087–86,429 cpm (to measure T and B cell function)
Concanavalin A	35,275–176,670 cpm (to measure T cell function)

Note: These tests are performed by measuring the incorporation of titrated thymidine into lymphocytes stimulated with the mitogens listed. Cpm indicates the amount of thymidine incorporation. Unstimulated lymphocytes usually incorporate <1,000 cpm.

TABLE B-8. FLOW CYTOMETRY FOR CD4/CD3/CD8 (IMMUNE COMPETENCE PANEL)

	Normal range (%)	Absolute numbers
Anti-CD3 (pan T cell markers)	54–87	650–1,770
Anti-CD4 (helper/inducer T cell markers)	32–60	400–1,175
Anti-CD8 (cytotoxic/suppressor T cell markers)	13–43	145–820

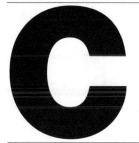

Sample Schedule for Perennial Aqueous Immunotherapy

Jill A. Poole

SAMPLE BUILDUP FOR WEEKLY IMMUNOTHERAPY AND SUGGESTED METHODS FOR LABELING DILUTIONS

Dilution	Volume (mL)
1:1000	0.05
Number 4 or green	0.1
	0.3
	0.5
1:100	0.05
Number 3 or blue	0.1
	0.2
	0.3
	0.4
	0.5
1:10	0.05
Number 2 or yellow	0.05
	0.1
	0.2
	0.3
	0.35
	0.4
	0.45
	0.5
1:1 Maintenance concentrate	0.05
Number 1 or red	0.1
	0.15
	0.2
	0.25
	0.3
	0.35
	0.4
	0.45
	0.5

Note: Dilutions expressed as volume/volume from the maintenance concentrate vaccine.
Reprinted from reference 25, with permission.

Index

Page numbers followed by *t* indicate tables; numbers followed by *f* indicate figures.